ENDURING

ENDURING

*A Story of Love, Dementia,
and Lessons Learned*

DONNA LARKIN

ENNISTYMON PRESS

Published by Ennistymon Press
www.donnalarkin.com

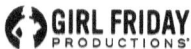

Edited and designed by Girl Friday Productions
www.girlfridayproductions.com

Design: Paul Barrett
Project management: Sara Spees Addicott and Laura Dailey

ISBN (paperback): 979-8-9889525-0-3
ISBN (ebook): 979-8-9889525-1-0

Library of Congress Control Number: 2023920610

First Edition

CONTENTS

PREFACE

My caregiver friends and I worked as hard as we could, some for a decade, to learn what we needed to know to competently care for our loved ones with dementia. Most of us went to classes and support-group meetings, read books, and networked with knowledgeable caregiving veterans who were willing to share their expertise and experiences.

After our husbands passed away one by one, we voiced a common frustration: the knowledge and experience we had amassed was going to be lost. Then the pandemic took hold. With plenty of solitude and time on my hands, I had the opportunity to at least pass on the story of one caregiver.

I began the project by printing out emails with detailed descriptions of my husband's condition—emails I'd written over seven or so years to family and friends. Then I pulled together the diary and calendars I hadn't been able to bring myself to throw away. And I printed text messages I'd sent over nearly ten years. The resulting book is an abbreviated nine-year journal, the story of one person's approach to and efforts at full-time, primary caregiving, or at least of the events and caregiving aspects that, at the time, I thought were important enough to document. Since I didn't record the stories of other family members and friends who were also affected by my husband's dementia, their stories are not included here except where they intersected with my own story. And so, this caregiving chronicle is skewed toward a wife's perspective.

The events and challenges that were on my mind at the time I wrote an email, note, or calendar entry formed the basis for this book. Even though I may have missed documenting some events, I am sure new caregivers will be left with a strong sense of what it took for me to be a dementia caregiver for my husband. On the flip side, a story or two may seem a bit too detailed for the casual reader, especially around the topic of hygiene. However, my target audience is current, active caregivers who may need the included information.

Although I'm hoping that my story will help to prepare caregivers, I am not a medical or legal expert. Nothing in this book is intended to be professional advice. The pages here simply tell my story of caregiving and describe the things you may feel I did right and the things I could have done better. I sincerely hope that every caregiver finds many other sources of information about the type of dementia afflicting her loved one and finds advice from many different types of experts. The wider I ventured with my research, the better prepared I felt as a caregiver.

The caregivers I came to know over the years desperately needed help, and most didn't get anywhere near enough of it. My heart goes out to those struggling right now to care for their loved ones. This book is dedicated to you. Know that I send prayers your way every day.

INTRODUCTION

During the hot summer, I developed a habit of visiting the TCBY frozen-yogurt shop near my house once a week. I'd order a cup of soft golden vanilla with chocolate chips on top, then sit on a bench on the shop's front patio to watch the traffic go by as I savored the cool sweetness. For the first time in two decades, my evenings were used as I saw fit, and what I wanted—needed—was to remember how to enjoy my life again. I had bought a little patio home just a few months earlier and worked with a friend to renovate it. Now, on weekend mornings, I took long walks on the greenbelt before it got too hot, and on Saturday nights, I learned line dancing with girlfriends. I was trying to find my way as a single woman.

One really hot evening in mid-July, a handsome gentleman sat down on the bench next to mine. Ostensibly watching a car drive by, I observed him out of the corner of my eye. He had an air about him, a "man's man" way of carrying himself as some men do, as if they are in a cologne or tequila ad in *GQ*.

When I looked in his direction, he smiled wide, then said, "Hello. Quite a hot day today, wasn't it?"

His smile accentuated deep dimples, which made me want to smile, too. I don't remember exactly what I said about the weather in reply, but I do remember that soon we were venturing beyond small talk, speaking openly about our professions, his retirement, our respective kids, and what we had been doing with our summers so far. I was mesmerized by his sparkling blue eyes and immediately drawn to his particular magnetism. Actually, he made my heart flutter.

I'd been divorced for a year and a half, and I savored my freedom as much as I savored every bite of that frozen yogurt. I was intent on protecting my new life, my new sense of peace. For the first time in as long as I could remember, I was content. Life was far from perfect, but it was good enough. Still, I really took my time that day finishing my yogurt and was sadder than usual to see the white cardboard bottom of the cup. If I were to be honest with myself, I would have to admit that I hated leaving the conversation, that I wanted to stay and talk to this man, this Lee with the bright blue eyes. I was good at hiding those feelings—even from myself—and put on a big smile as I put my spoon in the cup and got to my feet.

"So," Lee said casually, "I know that this is probably presumptuous, having just met you on a bench outside a frozen-yogurt shop, of all places." He stopped to laugh, then continued, "I know I am being a bit forward, but I was wondering . . . would you consider going to dinner with me?"

He was giving me an awesome grin that accentuated those crazy dimples, which made him so endearing. It was as if I were under a spell—or maybe that was an excuse for why I said yes. I had a strong sense that I could trust him, but then I got a jab in the gut and remembered my oath to avoid any entanglements. I quickly told him that I wasn't interested in a relationship right now and that he would need to agree that this was a one-time-only date. He just smiled a big smile.

On our first date at the Chart House, Lee opened the passenger door and offered his arm. It had been a very long time since a man had done that for me. As we walked toward the restaurant, I again observed him out of the corner of my eye. He was trim, with broad shoulders. His dark hair and gray sideburns and mustache were perfectly trimmed, and his clothes fit beautifully. In fact, his tie was knotted so perfectly, I thought it had to be one of those fake cheater ties with an elastic band that slips under the collar. (I learned later that he really did knot his ties perfectly.) I remember thinking that, with those deep dimples, this man strongly resembled a younger Sean Connery.

Lee had a reservation, so we walked right through the lobby and past the crowd waiting for tables. The host seated us by a window, in a room dimly lit by the candles on each cloth-covered table. Outside, cottonwood trees lined the river, creating a dreamy, dusk-muted backdrop. As we sipped our wine, he turned the conversation back to me, acting as though he was completely taken with everything I had to say. The time flew by.

After parking in my driveway, Lee again opened the car door for me and walked me to my front door.

"Can I call you in a couple of days, to go out for coffee?"

"Yes, of course," I said, smiling at him but not reaching for his hand or leaning in to give him a hug. I just couldn't. Lee must have been able to tell I needed the distance and didn't lean in either.

From my front window, I watched this mysterious man return to his car, walking tall yet with grace. For two hours, I had felt like a princess. He had made me feel like a princess. *Oh my gosh,* I thought with a sigh. *Who is this guy?*

During the next six months, on the days when we didn't ride bikes, cruise on his boat, go to plays or concerts, take picnics to the park, or have dinners out, I'd work out on my elliptical at 7:00 p.m. like clockwork, then take a shower and listen for the phone call that always came at around 9:00 p.m.

Lee's voice was deep and clear, a radio announcer's voice, and he was really funny. He told stories about the places he'd been, the people he had met, and the amazing experiences he'd had in Iowa, California, Texas, Florida, Massachusetts, Illinois,

England, Spain, Greece, Turkey, and Iran. He described his work, first in weather forecasting and then in a solar program, working to calculate the probability of future solar activity while stationed in observatories around the world.

Lee called me "the Blonde" in a teasing tone and made jokes about how I fit the stereotype of the excitable, impulsive blonde. Yet he teased in a way that let me know he was attracted to those qualities, that he found me intriguing. He'd also laid out the evidence on why he thought I was smart and capable and told me he was proud of my recent accomplishments, ending nearly every call by saying how lucky he was to have met me. I'd hang up feeling appreciated and respected for who I was, even my airheaded side. I had never talked for so long with anyone on the phone. After some months had passed, Lee started speaking sweet nothings in Spanish and Greek and mailing me beautiful love letters when he traveled. The effects of those calls washed into my days, giving me a new confidence at work.

I had completed facilitating a "business process redesign" for two departments of an organization in town and then was assigned as interim manager for one of those areas. The organization was converting to a new enterprise-wide information-technology system. It was a huge project, and the hours were brutal, with frequent twelve-hour days, often seven days a week. Lee picked me up from work midday once or twice a week.

He advised, "You need time away from work, or you'll burn out. I'm sure all of your coworkers need breaks and take them, too. You can't allow yourself to become a slave to your job, or you'll end up hating it . . ." And so on until he wore me down.

I'll never forget walking out of the old brick building and down the sidewalk that bordered a permit-only parking lot. I'd always see Lee first, waiting patiently in his car as it idled at the curb on the other side of the street, with a serious look on his face as he tried to catch sight of me. Once he spotted me waiting to cross at the corner, the widest smile would light up his face. Lee always had a nearby restaurant in mind and made sure I got back to work within my self-imposed ninety-minute time limit.

Every so often, I'd receive a large, unusual flower arrangement delivered by Jack's Flower to my office, with a handwritten card attached that usually had a few lines about what a jewel I was in his life. I teased Lee, calling him "my Sean," as in Sean Connery, and he teased me right back by signing those romantic cards simply as "Sean." None of my coworkers' boyfriends or husbands sent them flowers, and the women naturally became curious about the man who was responsible for these huge bouquets. When Lee started calling me his princess, I really felt like one.

Yet despite all of Lee's wonderful qualities, I decided to break up with him after six months. I was sure that he was still grieving his late wife's death from cancer two years earlier. At the time, I had not yet experienced or been compelled to learn about the grieving process. Obviously, I thought, Lee wasn't ready for a relationship. And I suspected I wasn't either. The final straw, however, was Lee's age. Eventually he divulged that he was sixty-eight—much older than he looked and acted. Our twenty-year age gap scared the heck out of me, and, to be honest, it was a little embarrassing. I had overheard a few snide comments about our "May-December relationship."

I knew that if I tried to break up with Lee in person, I'd never go through with it, so I sent him a "Dear John" letter. He honored my wishes by not contacting me in response, and I missed him. Badly. Every day. Regardless, I held strong, reminding myself of the very reasonable reasons for the breakup, telling myself that I'd done what was best, that I'd ripped that bandage off and now I just had to wait for the sting to fade away.

That wait lasted six months. After an especially tough week at work, I couldn't stop myself from calling Lee. To my surprise, he didn't bring up the "Dear John" letter at all and offered to meet me for coffee.

Sitting down in front of him, I blurted out, "I'm sorry. It's incredibly selfish of me to ask for your time after . . . everything. After treating you badly."

"Donna," he said, taking my hand, "I don't want to hear another word about the time apart. You needed it."

I gazed into his blue eyes as I spilled out my problems. My work project wasn't going well, and one of my coworkers had suffered a heart attack from the stress.

"I can feel myself going down, too," I said. "I'm working as an interim manager, and while keeping the department running, I'm also training the staff on the new system. Every day I find broken accounts, accounts where the new system is not cross-referencing correctly, and then I have to manually go into the system to correct the links within those accounts."

What I didn't say was that I had realized that Lee had been there for me months ago, in a way that no one else had. He was the calm and the peace at the end of the day, the cheering section, the gas in my emotional tank. During the last few months, instead of spending my evenings with him, I'd been going home to an empty house every night, feeling exhausted yet too stressed out to sleep.

"I'm sorry," I said again, "about all of this whining—"

"Donna," he said, taking my hand again. "Are you training the folks on the new system and fixing the accounts as best you can?"

"Yes," I said, "but the people I'm training look to me for answers that I don't have, and the customers affected by the broken accounts are worked up by the time they reach me."

"Well, it sounds like you're doing everything humanly

possible. The problems are not your fault, but you're making sure they don't impact the customers any longer than absolutely necessary. There's nothing else that anyone could do. Be proud of your effort and proud that you care. Take breaks with the knowledge that you are doing all you can to help."

By the time we'd finished our coffee, I felt that I could deal with tomorrow's challenges, and I had to admit to myself that this was it. Despite the age difference, our connection was undeniable. We were inseparable from then on.

After a year or so, Lee asked me to sit down at his kitchen table one afternoon so we could talk.

"If you want to end the relationship, now is the time," he told me.

That ship has sailed, I thought as he continued.

"I have been thinking about the fact that, if we continue on, our age difference is going to become a real issue at some point. We have to face the possibility that you could be spending years in the future caring for me, and I . . ."

He paused; his uncertainty was just so foreign. "I don't want to do that to you. But on the other hand, I also want to be with you for . . . well, forever."

Lee was strong, surefooted and clearsighted, the most confident man I'd ever known. I just couldn't picture him any other way. I certainly couldn't imagine his being infirm and requiring my care. I remember thinking that I'd rather have a few happy years with Lee than a lifetime of missing him.

After a minute or two, I gave Lee my opinion about our relationship. "You know that I've been under the care of a cardiologist for almost twenty years. It could just as easily be me who needs your care someday. Let's not worry about tomorrow. I want to be with you, too," I told him.

We never revisited that decision. Lee often said that it was fate that caused us to meet at the yogurt shop; I thought God's hand was in our meeting. We both were certain as could be that we were meant to be together. It was easy to ignore snide remarks about our age difference; they never could pierce our happiness bubble.

CHAPTER 1

2000S

From the very beginning of our courtship, Lee and I thoroughly enjoyed our lives together: biking, boating, picnicking, going to concerts and plays, walking the greenbelt, traveling, and gardening. Most of all, Lee loved to go out to eat. If someone could truly "live for" something, then he lived for going out to restaurants. In fact, if it were up to him, we'd go out to eat every day.

Brunch had always been Lee's favorite outing. Each Sunday, he practically ran out of church once the service was over so he could beat the brunch rush at whichever restaurant he had already chosen. We tried most new establishments within a month or two of their opening. I have to admit, I did love having a leisurely brunch, especially during the seven or eight months a year when it was possible for us to dine al fresco. Lee always ordered the same thing—two eggs over easy, hash browns, toast, and bacon—but he made a point to seek out places for me that offered unique veggie omelets, quiches, and pastries.

On Friday nights, we often went to Casa Mexico. Lee ordered picadillo enchiladas and chatted in Spanish with the staff while I tried fajitas, chili rellenos, tamales, or the nightly special. At his favorite Greek restaurant, Romio's, Lee casually conversed with the Greek owner while eagerly waiting for his pastitsio to be served. Of course, we'd go by TCBY for frozen yogurt at least twice a week.

We were happy.

THE FIRST CHALLENGE

After six or seven years of marriage, Lee started having trouble sleeping through the night. This was a sad turn of events, given how much we both looked forward to lying next to each other at the end of the day. Nothing made me feel safer or more loved than resting my head on Lee's shoulder and feeling his arm around me, pulling me into him. As the insomnia worsened, he developed a routine of waking up in the wee hours, which woke me up, too. At a routine medical appointment, my primary-care physician asked me if I was tired—apparently sleep deprivation was written on my face or in my body language.

"Perhaps you could move into a spare bedroom?" he asked.

When he saw my face drop, he added, "Just until the cause of Lee's sleeplessness can be figured out."

Lee asked me to ignore the doctor's advice, but unless I quit my job and took daily naps, it would be impossible. Then the sleeplessness got worse. Lee became unable to sleep for hours at a time. Some nights he got only two or three hours of sleep, and that caused him great anxiety.

"I just have to find a fix," he kept saying.

During the day, he looked like a sleepwalking zombie. Lee's doctor ordered a study in a sleep lab, which resulted in a severe apnea diagnosis. The wires and monitors hooked up to him during that one night in the lab revealed that he had stopped breathing multiple times every minute. The sleep specialist, a pulmonologist, was shocked by how often during the night Lee was oxygen deprived. A CPAP breathing machine was ordered, but Lee got so frustrated whenever he tried to sleep with its mask on that he eventually refused to even talk about using it. Short of cooperating with the CPAP, there was nothing more that could be done about the apnea.

To endure those middle-of-the-night waking hours, Lee developed a habit of watching TV in bed. Even though I was now sleeping in the next room, the sound from the television woke me up, which defeated the whole purpose of sleeping separately. A year or so into the struggle, I found a set of wireless headphones that worked with our bedroom television. Lee thought they were a Godsend! Now he could turn up the volume as loud as he wanted without worrying about waking me.

DIAGNOSIS

In the summer of 2009, Lee and I took a trip to his hometown in southwest Iowa to visit extended family. Initially, there'd been some confusion about whether we'd go to Lincoln, Nebraska, to see Lee's brother or whether he would visit us at the house of their sister in Iowa. Lee and his brother went back and forth on the phone, trying to get the plans worked out. In the end, his brother and sister-in-law made the drive to see us. We had a great time together.

It was revealed during the visit that his brother had Alzheimer's disease, which came as a huge shock, especially since, to me, he seemed fine overall. However, after we spent a couple of hours together, I noticed that he seemed to get very weary. His wife told me that she did all of the driving now, too. Immediately after everyone posed for a group picture under the big tree in the front yard, he got into the passenger seat of his car, looking exhausted. Lee's brother died three years later.

The day after we flew back home, Lee told his son and daughter-in-law at brunch, with genuine sadness and a little frustration, that we hadn't been able to see his brother while in Iowa. I knew in a flash that there was something wrong with my husband and immediately wondered if Lee had experienced a stroke during the trip. I pushed him to see a neurologist, and Lee agreed to go along with the examination, I think in order to prove me wrong. Deep down, I assumed that he would easily be able to overcome any possible diagnosis.

In the exam room, I sat beside my husband as the neurologist went through a cognitive function test. I recognize now that it was a test called the Mini-Mental State Exam.

"I want you to remember three words," the doctor began. "Ball. Tree. Penny. Got it? Ball, tree, penny."

Lee smiled wide and nodded; then the two chatted casually about the local football team. Five minutes later, the doctor asked Lee to repeat back the three words; then to tell him the name of the current president, the day of the week, and the name of the town we were in; then to subtract seven from one hundred and then again from the answers twice more; and then to touch his nose with his index finger. Lee was patient and answered the questions as if they were part of a game.

Everything seemed fine to me. Yet to be honest, I was so confident that Lee didn't have dementia, I hadn't really paid attention to his answers to the doctor's questions. At the end of the examination, I expected the doctor to say that there was nothing to worry about. Instead, the neurologist told us out of the blue that Lee probably had Alzheimer's disease. Lightning struck my heart in that room, and I did all I could to avoid showing it.

"I'll order a brain scan and blood work to rule out other causes," the doctor said while entering into Lee's chart a prescription for a drug that he explained might lessen some symptoms for a while. "But there's no medication yet that can forestall the progression of the disease."

I glanced at Lee. His expression was unreadable. I did my best to keep my face neutral, too.

The neurologist had a reputation for being the best in the area; we trusted his opinion. Lee left the office with a tentative diagnosis, and I left with a book that the doctor handed directly to me: *The 36-Hour Day*. I didn't realize at the time why the doctor had intentionally handed the book to me . . . that it falls to the primary loved one to figure out how to best adjust our lives in order to cope with the disease. It would be up to me to help Lee deal with the symptoms as they appeared. I was completely ignorant about what was to come and my role.

We walked silently back to the car. On the drive home, Lee chatted about the doctor's opinion of the football team's chances that year. I knew that my husband had to be just as shocked by the diagnosis as I was. *Maybe he's buying time to let it sink in?* He had told me early in our marriage that, to him, the absolute worst way "to go" would be to lose his mental faculties. This had to be devastating news for him.

Walking into the house, I put down my purse and blurted out without any introduction, "I meant it when I vowed for better or for worse, in sickness and in health. I will stand by your side, no matter what." I exhaled deeply—I had broached the subject. Now I waited to hear Lee's reaction to the news. He just smiled and turned on the television.

DENIAL

Lee never mentioned the diagnosis, and while it seems unbelievable to me now, I put the topic out of my mind after a day or two. I was married to a twenty-seven-year veteran of the US

Air Force, a man who had won an award for developing a system to track and calculate the probability of solar flares, who was fluent in multiple languages and completely at ease with traipsing all over the globe. This was a brilliant, logical man, as strong as anyone I'd ever known. Even with the age difference, he rode circles around me on his bike. Lee cranked his boat down to the water at the marina and back up onto the trailer as if it weighed nothing. Years earlier, I'd been so sick I could barely walk, and he had effortlessly lifted my dead weight from the floor and carried me across the house to put me to bed. I couldn't believe that he could be brought down by anything. It just wasn't possible for me to picture my husband as disabled.

Lee still called me at work at lunchtime to tell me he missed me; every day he greeted me at the door when I got home. Once in a while, he'd call me from a restaurant to tease me with "Guess where I am . . ." Lee loved to drive, and we still took leisurely Sunday rides along country roads, stopping every now and then so I could take photos of the bright native wildflowers in bloom or of old farmhouses and barns that had views of low mountains in the distance, a clear blue sky as background, and wild tousled-looking pastures as foreground. Rusted barbed-wire fences still defined ownership of long-unused acreages, with barn roofs and upper siding scattered on the ground around their foundations. We still sipped cups of coffee over the newspaper on Saturday mornings before he whisked me off to a restaurant for brunch.

At the beginning of our marriage, my children were all working or going to college out of state. Lee and I had enjoyed spending most of our spare time together. Now it was almost as if he craved spending time with me. My routine changed gradually, almost imperceptibly, until my chores and hobbies and social life were squeezed into small slices of time wedged here and there. I hardly noticed—I so enjoyed my life with my husband. His speech was clear, and, as far as I could tell, his thinking was sound. The man I had married was still walking through life right alongside me, and our relationship, our day-to-day, felt normal, the same as it had always been. *Lee is too smart for dementia,* I suspected.

Then I made the mistake of mentioning the diagnosis to a coworker who had lost a husband to dementia.

"You're in for a hellish future," she said.

Her pitiful look and body language said even more. After that, no matter what I was doing during the day, a dark sense of foreboding hung over me. My period of denial was over.

MENTORING

Lee had pushed hard for us to live in his house, which was double the size of mine. Instead, I wanted to move into a smaller home that would be easier to keep up, one without such a large backyard. Lee argued that he'd moved more than enough while in the Air Force, and that after finally getting to live for a few years in one place, he felt he had roots at last. I could empathize and thought it would be almost cruel of me to uproot someone who'd spent a lifetime in temporary housing—and especially selfish given that he had made every one of those moves on behalf of my country. So, I had conceded and moved in with him. When I began making plans to sell my house, Lee advised me to rent it out instead.

"You don't have much equity, and realtor fees will eat that up," he explained.

Even though I wouldn't break even right away, between the rent proceeds in and the mortgage, taxes, and homeowner's and flood insurances out, he told me that my house would eventually build a good retirement fund for me.

"You'll want to make extra principal payments and hire a property manager, so you don't have to worry about finding decent renters," he added.

I never would have thought to hang on to the house or to get a property manager without Lee's advice and was grateful for his suggestion when I sold it twenty years later. My husband was savvy about finances, as he was about so many other topics. I just couldn't see him as otherwise. So, I was shocked six months after Lee's Alzheimer's diagnosis when I opened a letter from our credit union saying that our checking account was overdrawn. It was a first. I immediately panicked, assuming someone had nefariously accessed the account and emptied it. When I went through the checkbook and our online banking information, I didn't find any strange or unexpected debits. I dug a little deeper into the checkbook's entries for the last two months and realized that my husband had made a $1,000 mathematical error in the check register.

Lee read the overdraft letter, examined the checkbook, and then looked off into the distance. I expected him to promise to be more careful from now on, or to give some reasonable explanation for the error, or simply to say, "I'm only human."

Instead, he said, "You should take over."

This was the first time Lee had acknowledged any limitation. I hadn't seen any issues coming and felt blindsided and stressed out taking over our finances. I began keeping an Excel spreadsheet so I could track every transaction to the penny, and Lee took on the mentor role in earnest. He encouraged me, occasionally looking through the checkbook, going through the monthly statements, monitoring our online bank account, and giving me advice. Eventually, I built confidence and relaxed, and so did he. Then Lee took me to an appointment with his financial adviser and arranged for her to explain his investments to me as he looked on. At that appointment, they completed the investment firm's own power of attorney form, which would be required if I ever had to take any action with Lee's investments at the firm. A year later, Lee's younger daughter-in-law emailed me a copy of our state's financial power of attorney form and durable power of attorney for health care form and explained that Lee's son thought it was very important for his dad to get those generic forms completed as soon as possible. I didn't realize at the time how critical all of this advice would turn out to be.

SUPPORT

The overdraft felt like a wake-up call and spurred me to call my state's Commission on Aging office to ask about local family-caregiver resources and classes. The agency's receptionist recommended their Powerful Tools for Caregivers class.

"Please sign me up," I asked, then anxiously waited two weeks for the class to begin.

Would Lee feel funny if he knew I was attending a caregiver's class and worry that I saw him as infirm? The class ended up being held during the lunch hour, so I sidestepped that issue. I hoped that this class would make it possible for me to meet other caregivers, hear about various caregiving recommendations, and learn a little about what to expect, but ultimately, I discovered that the class wasn't about dementia caregiving per se. It was about caregiver stress and self-care. I was drawn to show up for the class anyway—if for nothing else than to hear about the other caregivers' challenges. The class ended up providing me with all sorts of information that came out as the attendees chatted, yet it turned out that the most helpful outcome of the class was meeting the instructor, Jerri.

Jerri was a perky, barely five-foot-three, funny, and confident woman in her midfifties who wore dark lip liner and a 1960s-style blonde bouffant hairdo, which I suspected might be a wig. I couldn't stop staring at that lip liner. As a former administrator at a memory-care facility in California, she had plenty of wisdom beyond the course's official material to share with the class. I soon realized she was one of the most endearing people I'd ever met. After a few classes, Jerri invited me to join a new, by-invitation-only dementia support group that she was forming.

"I'll be hosting a dinner for the group in a couple of weeks," she revealed.

Jerri hugged me at her front door, then proudly showed me the dining-room table's decorations. It looked like a Hobby Lobby bomb had gone off on the table, with dainty hand-painted plaster statuettes, Fabergé-knockoff eggs, pastel plates, Easter-themed napkins, and bunches of brightly colored tulips in vases.

"Welcome!" she said as she gave me her infectious smile. I'd never seen anything like that dining-room table before, I remarked. She was so proud!

The windows were open, spring was in the air, and "easy listening" music was wafting in from the living room as Jerri led me to the kitchen, where she introduced me to four of the eight other invitees, those who'd arrived before I had. They were all about my age or a touch older and welcomed me with bright smiles, as though we were at a party. As the others arrived, we nibbled on classic appetizers—guacamole and chips and spinach-artichoke dip with crostini—and talked about whether we worked and, if so, what kind of work we did. From the outside, I'm sure it looked like the warm-up to a wedding shower or some other ladies-only social function.

Keeping up the party pretense got tiring really quickly. Before we'd had our fill of the appetizers, the mood quickly shifted, as if everyone simultaneously conceded that we were over trying to put on happy faces. It was almost as if Jerri had said, "All right, let's go around the room and give a two-minute rundown on when your husband was diagnosed, how it was discovered, and how he is doing now."

The conversation instantly went deep. When we compared our husbands' diagnoses dates, I realized that most husbands were much further along in their diseases than Lee. I was hopeful I could learn from the others' experiences. Betsy told the group that her husband was sweet and compliant but required more and more help. Maureen's husband had started to fight her on everything. Pat talked about how tired her husband was all the time. Mickey had recently returned from a trip on which her husband had slipped out of their hotel room in the middle of the night, resulting in an impromptu search party. Ruth's husband had passed away a year ago; she graciously provided compassionate support. Jerri's husband did not have dementia, but she added comments based on her professional experience. Jerri seemed to understand exactly what each of us was going through. Nothing surprised her.

Those in the group with yearslong experience with dementia caregiving provided sage advice for the newbies. Some of the details were hard to hear, but we were drunk on the fact that we could talk so openly with others in similar situations. We had an instant comradery, an immediate simpatico, that made me think of my father and uncles, who had fought in World War II and the Korean War. They never spoke about their combat experiences with family but were drawn to the VFW hall, where they could commiserate with other combat vets. At that moment, I understood those men in a way I never had before. I realized that the women of this new caregiver support group were homebound soldiers in a losing battle.

I had an epiphany at that first support-group meeting as I listened to each woman's story: no one—not doctors, professional caregivers, family, friends, or me—could predict the trajectory of Alzheimer's disease, not how it would change its victims or how the disease would affect their caregivers.

By listening to the others, I realized that dementia's mani-festation is unique to every person with the disease, and so every caregiver's experience is different. I left with an *Alice in Wonderland* feeling, disoriented yet not completely lost. There were a million unknowns on the road ahead, but these fellow travelers were just a phone call away, ready to provide support to each other. The group would realize over time just how blessed we were and how important it was to have that safety net.

CHAPTER 2

2012

Lee was diagnosed with Alzheimer's disease in 2009, but I really didn't notice much of an effect from the disease until a couple of years later. By 2012, there were several dementia symptoms and behaviors that were beginning to have an impact on Lee's life, although that impact was hidden from most. I read that very intelligent people are adept at hiding their dementia because they have the bandwidth to slip quite a bit cognitively yet still be sharper than most people around them. That was my husband. He was very good at covering his tracks and hiding the evidence when he was around other people, especially if they were with him for just a couple of hours at a time every so often.

Lee was hiding the dementia from himself, too. Years later, once the signs were undeniable, I realized that he was actually unable to recognize his own Alzheimer's symptoms. I learned that this lack of awareness of an impairment is called anosognosia and affects up to 81 percent of those with Alzheimer's disease. It's a neurological condition believed to be caused by damage to the part of the brain that affects a person's perception of his own illnesses. Anosognosia leads people with dementia to believe that they are normal and able to do as much as always. Until the week he died, Lee was authentically fighting to convince people, including me, that he wasn't affected at all by the Alzheimer's disease.

THE REGULAR

As Lee's dementia progressed, so did his intense desire to eat out. If I tried to skip a day to work on a project or clean the house, he kept harping on me the way a fifteen-year-old boy might be prone to do when wanting the latest video game. The urge to go out to a restaurant was so strong by 2012, it completely took over Lee's focus every morning.

It didn't entirely make sense to me that Lee craved eating out, because by three years after his diagnosis, the entire experience was rife with struggles. For one, the breadth of the menu choices and descriptions overwhelmed him. As he got that pained look on his face while frantically trying to make sense of the menu, I'd quickly scan mine to find three or so options I knew he'd like and then list them out loud. When he heard something that was appealing, he'd immediately stop me, announce his choice, and look down at the table, concentrating on remembering. As soon as the waitperson came to the table, I ordered for both of us, and Lee looked visibly relieved. I knew it was considered unconventional for a woman to order for a man, and doing so made me feel very uncomfortable, like a "pushy" wife. Regardless, I continued to order for us, and Lee became more and more appreciative of my initiative.

My husband was a traditional guy, so he naturally reached for the check as soon as it arrived, immediately pulling out his debit card. In the early years of our marriage, Lee could do all sorts of computations in his head—he had used calculus daily at work for decades, after all. Now he had trouble calculating a simple tip and strained to keep me from knowing. He might leave a fifteen-dollar tip for an eighteen-dollar breakfast or three dollars for a thirty-five-dollar dinner, and then usually forgot to sign the slip.

In fact, he'd often point to the charge slip and say, "What is this line for? Am I supposed to sign it? Why?"

By 2012, I was attempting to shore up Lee's payment process without his catching on. I'd sneak my signature onto charge slips if needed. When he undertipped, I'd change the amount or tuck cash into the check presenter. Just before we left, I'd make sure that Lee took his debit card. If not, I'd slip it into my purse and sneak it back into his wallet as he was going to bed. I wasn't that good at deception, and when Lee caught me taking any of these measures to help, he'd stomp off to the car and stay angry for at least an hour.

On the other hand, at the Griddle, we were able to sidestep most of these restaurant struggles. I suspected that the manager, Grant, had some experience with dementia, because he anticipated Lee's needs masterfully, in a way that avoided embarrassment and conveyed compassion without condescension. Grant would boom out a big greeting to Lee as he walked through the door and see him to "our table." Lee would beam and fire back little bantering jokes toward Grant. This interchange seemed to make Lee feel welcomed and accepted.

Grant or his staff took Lee's order by simply asking, "You want the regular?" so he could just say, "Sure!" and feel like he blended in with the "normal" patrons.

Grant could always sense if Lee became a little bored or stressed and knew how to gently kid Lee to get a rise and chuckle out of him. Lee loved to sit in the sunshine that came beaming through the restaurant's two walls of floor-to-ceiling windows and work on the crossword with me while waiting for our orders to be delivered. Grant and his staff noticed when Lee was concentrating on the crossword and quietly filled our coffees without interrupting. The check was always surreptitiously dropped in front of me, so I could quickly pay it while Lee pretended not to notice. Those Griddle brunches seemed to feed my husband's soul and are some of my happiest memories from those years.

By 2012, Lee was exhausted by dinnertime, so we never went out in the evening. In fact, dinners at home became a real struggle. Soon after I placed his dinner plate before him, there would be a spill or some kind of turmoil, which reminded me of the times when my children were young and overtired. I'd make light of Lee's accidents, trying to keep the situation from becoming a damper on how well he ate.

Lee balked at any food from other cultures that he had formerly loved—he had especially liked Greek, Spanish, and Mexican food—but now automatically disliked any new recipes that I tried. I finally realized that he now preferred his childhood favorites, Iowa-style meat and potatoes. Yet even then, Lee ate robotically and often argued he wasn't hungry. Eventually, I found that if I kept Lee's attention engaged with storytelling, he would seem to eat on autopilot. Lee ate even better while sitting in front of the TV using a tray table. He'd focus on a show, usually sports or the news, and finish his meal without even noticing what was on the plate.

Dessert was a different story. "Vanilla ice cream with chocolate syrup caps off my evening just perfectly," he'd say. In talking with other support-group wives, I found that there was a common, intense need for sugar, especially chocolate, during late afternoons and evenings, almost as if there was no other way to get the energy they needed at those times. Lee absolutely had to have a sweet snack, like a brownie, every mid-afternoon, or he was unable to function.

Over the last fifteen years, Lee had enjoyed meals out much more than any other activity, yet now eating in or out was traumatic for Lee, as he fought fatigue, spills, and coordination problems. By 2012, mealtime had evolved into one of our biggest challenges.

INTERFERENCE

For many, many years, Lee's work took place at solar observatories located around the Mediterranean. He told me that his desks were always located near impact printers that were constantly spitting out satellite data and that was why he suffered from hearing loss and tinnitus. Eventually, Lee was fitted for hearing aids. These aids were so tiny that they were invisible to others. And they were very sophisticated, able to identify and tamp down ambient noise while accentuating nearby voices. Despite a real need for the hearing aids, Lee just couldn't get used to wearing them. I didn't know if it was the physical sensation or vanity or impatience with having to adjust the settings at first. All I knew was that he refused to wear them. I was disappointed and frustrated yet also sympathetic to the fact that Lee had an extra dose of male pride and an allergy to dependence. After he returned the aids for a refund, Lee never complained again about the tinnitus and seemed able to function well enough so that strangers had no clue he had a hearing problem.

Once the dementia took hold, Lee started getting upset in restaurants if there were loud conversations or music, especially the kind with repetitive lyrics or noticeable, reverberating beats. He would get a grouchy look on his face and fixate on the distraction, complaining loudly. From that point on, our outing would go down the tubes, and we'd have to rush whatever we were doing so we could leave as soon as possible. Even after leaving a location, the fallout continued; Lee was unable to regain his composure for the rest of the day. I saw a glimpse of a man I'd never known before, someone downright difficult to be around. The change was gut-wrenching for me. Sounds he found intolerable stole his wide smile and replaced it with a scowl and grousing. I heard from other caregivers whose husbands reacted in the same way to noise, especially to grandchildren's play. Even a nearby car's loud music while we sat at a traffic light threw Lee into a tailspin.

My grandkids were introduced to dementia at a Red Robin in 2012. I hadn't seen them in a month and was overjoyed to be sitting with the kids in a huge red booth, listening to their stories. Ben, seven years old, and Libby, nine years old, were taking turns telling Grandma and Grandpa all about school and Libby's latest swim meet. Then Ben took a turn excitedly describing his latest Legos building achievement. Two-year-old Eli was coloring on the children's menu and furtively glancing at a red balloon he hoped to get on our way out. The kids seemed to bask in our attention; this scene was the stuff of my earliest dreams about becoming a grandma.

After we ordered, the background music and conversations gradually ratcheted up as the restaurant became busier, when all of a sudden, it became too much for Lee. He abruptly got up and stormed out of the restaurant. I looked at the kids, their faces transformed from excited to worried.

"Is Grandpa mad at us?" Ben asked. That question felt like a punch to the gut.

"No, sweetheart," I said, trying to smile. "Grandpa's not mad at you. He's just not feeling well."

Before the waiter could serve our plates, I asked for five to-go boxes and the red balloon. In the car, the scowl on Lee's face kept my mouth shut, and the kids sat silently in the back seat. This wasn't the grandpa they knew and loved. From that point forward, the kids nearly always saw Lee at our home or at my daughter's home, where we could control the environment. Still, there would be times when Alzheimer's would obscure the true and loving spirit of my husband.

This kind of reaction to sound, or "interference," was common among my friends' husbands, as well. Most caregivers I knew understood that at some point, our husbands just couldn't cope with these normal, day-to-day sound annoyances. Most caregivers showed patience and empathy during times when the noise or commotion got to their husbands. On the other hand, a few caregivers acted as if their husbands still had control and were choosing to act out. This kind of interference became an issue in their relationships, causing the women to become extremely frustrated with and critical of their husbands. Dementia caregiving became really challenging to these caregivers at this point.

DRIVING

Lee's father had been a trusted mechanic in their small hometown and, at one time, part owner of a car dealership. Lee had been driving and working on cars from the time he was barely tall enough to see over a steering wheel and under a hood. By the time he was in high school, he knew how to independently keep his own clunker car running. As a result, Lee had an innate understanding of automotive mechanics.

When he was assigned to a small detachment at a solar observatory in Tehran, Lee shipped his car there and later had to overhaul its engine in a parking lot, with parts shipped by his brother. Soon his commanding officer recruited Lee to help keep his American car running, too. Although Lee no longer worked on cars by the time we met, it was a real plus that he had the know-how to deal with the dealership's mechanics when our vehicles needed maintenance. And so it seemed natural that Lee loved to drive. In years past, I'd watched him expertly navigate our vehicles over steep and narrow mountain roads, on city freeways, along forest-service roads at the edges of cliffs, and into slivers of parking spaces. He made it look easy. As a couple, we continued his tradition of Sunday drives, making our way through the countryside, taking in scenes straight out of Chuck Pinson or Thomas Moran paintings, exploring winding ribbons of blacktop country roads. I learned how to get around our entire valley as an outcome of these drives.

One afternoon in 2012, on a Sunday drive along a country road, Lee drove the car at least fifty miles per hour, ten over the limit, as we approached a four-way stop. *He isn't slowing,* I thought. *Is he going to stop?*

"Lee!" I yelled as he blew right through it. "There was a stop sign!"

"No, there wasn't," he said quietly, frowning at me.

The entire event was over in a second, but the shock was imprinted on my psyche. We had driven this road scores of times before without a problem. *What the heck happened? It's just one mistake,* I reassured myself, *something that anyone might have done.*

On the following Sunday, we were enjoying the ups and downs of a slightly hilly topography, on a road with an uneven dirt shoulder to our right and a faded yellow line down the middle. The scene was bucolic, except for an occasional new subdivision that dotted the landscape on the driver's side, the south side of the road. As Lee drove along this favorite stretch, I happened to look over and was surprised to see his head turned hard left. I waited and waited, and as I watched, Lee never returned his eyes to the road in front of the car. While the seconds ticked by, we drifted farther and farther right onto the dirt shoulder. Lee didn't seem to notice.

"Honey," I said, "why aren't you looking forward?"

"Oh." He immediately looked ahead. "I forgot I was driving."

I didn't comprehend. "Were you . . . sightseeing out the window?"

"Yes," Lee said quietly.

His demeanor became sheepish as he, too, absorbed what had just happened. For the rest of the drive, Lee kept his eyes glued to the road in front of him.

A few months later, as we were heading east to the other side of town, Lee merged our car onto the freeway but did not accelerate to match the traffic's pace. From my view, the speedometer read thirty miles per hour. Cars were zooming by us in flashes.

"Please, pick up the speed," I said, trying to keep the panic from my voice.

"What are you talking about?" Lee said. "I'm going the correct speed."

I wondered, *Does he know he is going too slowly but can't handle going any faster? Or does he actually have no sense of speed? Is he unable to read the speedometer or notice the cars zooming by?* I didn't think it was safe to press him, so I covertly clicked on the blinking hazard lights. Every time I turned around to check for cars coming up behind us, Lee harrumphed, as if I was overreacting. I prayed that the drivers would notice our emergency flashers, assume we were having car trouble, and go around. Luckily, the road wasn't too crowded with cars, and people easily navigated around us. The same thing happened three more times over the next couple of months.

I never discussed these driving issues with Lee while he was behind the wheel, afraid that I would upset him and cause a wreck. Once we were home, I did everything I could to convince him that it was time to take a driving test. Nothing worked. Every time I brought up the subject, Lee gave me the cold shoulder afterward, usually for the entire day. When it was clear that I was getting nowhere, I insisted that he allow me to drive, but he pushed past me to get into the driver's seat every time. I wouldn't give up, and Lee was furious. Dementia had now inserted itself into our marriage and was interfering with our peace. After having nightmares about our car crashing into that of some unlucky family, I wasn't going to give in, even if it meant struggles in our marriage.

Physicians were responsible for notifying my state's Department of Motor Vehicles anytime they deemed a resident of the state no longer competent to drive. At Lee's next appointments with his primary-care physician and his neurologist, I described the driving issues and begged them to report Lee's status to the DMV. Lee stormed out of the offices both times. Neither medical professional wanted to take responsibility for Lee's loss of driving privileges.

"Lee would be angry. He'd never come back to my office if I did that," they both said, almost as if they were reading from a script.

I had heard from other caregivers that physicians were commonly reluctant to do this kind of reporting, being averse to upsetting—and possibly losing—a patient. Besides, how did they know for sure that a patient was truly unable to drive?

So, that was that . . . My hands were tied. Then one day in 2012, Lee drove the car onto a busy two-lane freeway off-ramp that emptied onto a street near the mall. Our car started in the left lane, but as we rounded the ramp's curve to the left, it drifted into the right lane—and toward a car that was driving alongside us. I looked over and saw the front-seat passenger screaming. Thankfully, the driver was alert enough to slam on his brakes and make room for our car.

"What a jerk," Lee said when the driver honked his horn. He argued that he'd been in that right lane first, all along. This was the closest we'd come to a crash yet. I had to do something.

At a recent caregivers' support-group meeting, I'd heard

one of the wives talk about a new simulated driving test designed for people with brain injuries and dementia. It was offered at the local Elks Rehabilitation Hospital, in a laboratory with equipment that simulated a car. The lab had a video display in place of a windshield, and a dashboard, brake pedal, gas pedal, and steering wheel that were all hooked up to a computer. This simulation was lifelike, I heard, but the test was only administered to those with physicians' referrals. The day after our off-ramp near miss, I mailed letters describing the event to both the neurologist and the family-practice physician. "Lee is a danger to himself and others," I added, requesting a referral specifically for the specialized driving test at the Elks Hospital. Either putting my request in writing or recommending the new driving test made a difference. Within a couple of days, Lee had an appointment. I didn't dare give him advance notice of the test, and he was livid when I announced it was time to go.

"This is your chance to prove me wrong," I told him. "If you pass, I will never bring it up again."

Lee shot me the dirtiest look, as if his eyes could bore a hole in my chest.

"I'm driving there," he said.

I breathed a sigh of relief that at least he was complying with my request to move out to the car without putting up a fight. The huge, cavernous waiting area was crowded, but he didn't have to wait long. A technician called Lee's name and told me that they would be gone for at least one hour. I pulled out a book and tried to get myself emotionally ready for what would surely come. An hour and twenty minutes later, I looked up from my book to see Lee and the test technician walking toward me.

"It is imperative," the technician said loudly as they approached, "that your husband never get behind the wheel again."

I was afraid to look at Lee as she went on.

"His scores were about as low as I've ever seen. Do not allow this man to get behind the wheel of a car. Now that he's failed this test so badly, you will be held responsible if he harms anyone while driving. Do not allow this man to get behind the wheel of a car. I repeat: Do not allow this man to get behind the wheel."

"I won't," I said, feeling my cheeks turn red.

"That test proves nothing," Lee argued. "What does that test have to do with actual driving?"

As luck would have it, Lee's license expired the following week, and we had a flight booked for the following month, which meant he'd need a new, valid driver's license or state ID to get through TSA security. The day after the driving test, I drove us to the DMV. Thankfully, he didn't realize that he could have renewed his license without me and without taking a DMV driving test (except possibly an eyesight test). Lee literally threw his license at the clerk and said that he was being forced to turn it in.

The lady smiled kindly and said, "If it's due to a medical reason, you can get a free state identification card in its place."

"I have to turn it in because of Alzheimer's," he said.

I was absolutely floored to hear that admission out loud. Lee obediently moved to the side of the counter so the clerk could take a new picture for the ID. That picture is burned into my memory; it captured the very essence of Lee's emotions over losing his license. His face had the deepest furrowed brow and the most extreme scowl. After receiving his new ID card, he stormed out of the DMV building and got into the passenger seat of our car. It was one of our darkest days as a couple.

The driving habit was hard to break. Lee would often make a move toward the driver's side of the car, and I would have to remind him that he was uninsured now. With a look of utter disdain, he would concede the driver's seat to me. *That's Alzheimer's looking at me,* I'd tell myself, *not Lee.* Still, it broke my heart.

When we first got together, I was so excited that Lee loved to drive and was good at it. The support group talked about how much they had loved sitting beside their husbands as they confidently drove all over the country, too. I absolutely hated driving, and many of the wives echoed my sentiment. Now we had no choice. I did my best, but got us lost on a highway in Oregon and in a dangerous neighborhood in Phoenix. Lee would get impatient with me, expecting me to have his sense of direction and knowledge of the highways. I definitely wasn't celebrating that my husband had lost his license.

Lee was now housebound when I was at work, and within a few weeks, he descended into a real depression. I bought puzzles, Western novels . . . any form of entertainment I could find, but he didn't have the interest or the energy to participate. After I talked about Lee's depression with my manager, she suggested that I go into work early and take a long lunch break so I could get Lee out of the house middays. That was a great idea, I thought! The double commute was grueling but worth it when I saw Lee's face light up as I picked him up each day for lunch.

After lunch, I always laid a sweet snack on the table by his recliner and made sure that the television was set so he could watch his favorite classic television shows, like *Gunsmoke*, *Bonanza*, and *The Rifleman*, after I was gone. Yet it didn't matter what I did to set him up for the afternoon; he would always become forlorn and complain that he was "stuck at home" as I kissed him goodbye. I usually returned to work after lunch feeling down.

Lee soon forgot about taking the driving test itself, but he never, ever forgot who took him to the DMV to surrender his license.

NIGHTTIME

By 2012, I felt the need to help my husband with his night-time routine, and he loved the attention. If he would try to take off his shoes and socks without help, Lee lost his balance as he bent over, even if sitting on the bed. He often needed reminders to take nighttime medications and, about half the time, needed me to dole them out and watch to be sure he took them. Dirty clothes were placed in the hamper, Western paperbacks laid on top of his blankets, and bedding edges tucked under the mattress so he wouldn't trip if he got up during the night. He often needed help at times later in the night, too.

One night, I awoke to the sound of Lee thrashing and yelling. I raced into his room, turned on his light, and realized he was having a vivid nightmare.

"Lee!" I called out, trying to rouse him. "Honey!" I yelled even louder as I shook his shoulder a little.

Suddenly he snapped up into a sitting position, snatched hold of one of my wrists, and began fighting with all of his might, grunting and twisting my arm with lightning speed, so violently that it seemed like he broke it, all while he was still fast asleep.

"It's Donna!" I screamed over and over, crying out in pain. "It's me! Lee!"

He held fast for a couple of terrifying minutes before finally waking up enough to realize he should let go. I jumped back from the bedside, rubbing my wrist and trying to get my breathing under control. I immediately realized just how dangerous that situation could have been if he had not awakened when he did.

Lee shook his head. "I'm . . . I'm sorry," he said groggily. "I don't know what happened."

I never forgot from that night forward to keep a distance from his bed if Lee was fitful during sleep. His nightmares became a regular thing. I would turn on the light, shake the foot of the bed, and call to him loudly, trying to help him escape from the battles.

"Lee!! Wake up!! Honey, wake up!!"

His face would look determined, with teeth clenched as he grunted and punched and flailed around, putting his whole self into the fight. Sometimes, he'd touch something in the room and think it was part of his adversary's body. He fought with pillows, the headboard, and the objects on the nightstand. Some nights, he fought so hard he fell out of bed. One night I woke to a clanging and found Lee in a battle with his tall, very heavy brass lamp that was kept on the nightstand. He jerked the lamp into his forehead and tore open a gash. The lamp didn't fare much better. I replaced those brass lamps with lightweight plastic ones that turned out to be indestructible and much less dangerous.

After I told the neurologist about these nightmares, he adjusted the dose and timing of one of the Alzheimer's medications, which helped to cut way back on the frequency of the nightmares. Regardless, Lee required more and more help at night.

SUAVE AND DEBONAIR

Other than a neatly trimmed mustache, the Lee I'd first met had always been clean-shaven, with a tidy haircut. His shirtsleeves were sharply creased, and his ties and sweaters were perfectly coordinated. Everything fit him to a T, possibly because he had been convinced of the importance of a good fit by a London tailor who had custom-made a couple of sport coats and suits for Lee when he was stationed at Royal Air Force (RAF) Brize Norton outside Oxford, England. When I first met him, Lee's wardrobe was augmented every three months or so by an upscale store's saleswoman, who put together co-ordinated outfits for him and alerted him to sales in her men's department.

If I ever complimented him on an outfit, my husband would crack a joke about being "suave and debonair," but he would purposefully mispronounce the words as *swav-ey* and *de-bone-er.* His best friend, Bill, who had been stationed at Mountain Home Air Force Base for four years with Lee, would crack the same joke when given the opportunity. They always laughed with each other as if it were the first time they'd mis-pronounced the words, which tickled me, too. Bill was just as neat as Lee. I took their fastidiousness as an outcome of their respective decades-long military service.

But by 2012, Lee was too weary to run through his daily morning routine and started wearing crazy outfits. In winter, he might put on a light short-sleeved shirt, and in summer, he might reach for his favorite leather jacket. During the summer, I'd sometimes arrive home after work to find the doors and windows shut tight and the house as hot as a sauna. I soon learned to make sure the heater or AC was set for that after-noon's predicted conditions before I left for work each day. In the winter, I also draped a zip-up fleece sweatshirt over his recliner and laid a plush throw nearby before I left for work.

I knew that the former Lee would be mortified by this year's attire but didn't want to embarrass him; I ignored how he dressed. But if he was unshaven, or his hair was uncombed, or his clothes were inappropriate for the weather, or even if they were just mismatched, I started noticing that the public ignored or even avoided Lee. On the other hand, when he was dressed nicely like in years past, they showed him respect and interacted normally with him. So, I started getting more in-volved in Lee's grooming and laid out his next day's outfit as he got ready for bed each night. He seemed to like that, making jokes that I was dressing my Ken doll or that I was his valet.

Once Lee lost his driver's license, I drove him to the bar-bershop every four to six weeks. His barbershop was small, just one large room, with five chairs lining the left wall for waiting customers. Near the back, a potbellied stove kept the room toasty warm in the winter with logs chopped by Dewey, the owner and master fly fisherman. Mounted fish and fancy flies adorned the right wall over the sinks and mirrors. Lee had been a fly fisherman, too, and seemed proud that he could identify all of the fish on display. The taxidermied head of some kind of animal, an elk or deer or moose, looked down on the customers from the back wall. It gave me the creeps. Dewey opened the doors and windows to let in fresh air anytime the weather permitted.

I felt intimidated in this man's world. Occasionally, when Lee was having a good day, I'd leave him alone at the shop and run a quick errand. That way, he had some time alone with Dewey and the guys, and I didn't have to hang out there. More often than not, however, I'd end up sitting in one of the waiting chairs toward the back, if one was available, ostensibly reading but in actuality eavesdropping on the male conversations.

Dewey kept an eye on the parking lot, and when a familiar car pulled up, he'd give a quick lowdown on the new arrival.

"A great cop who retired ten years ago," he'd say.

Or: "That fellow lost his wife in a bad accident."

Or: "You'd never know it, but he's a real jerk to his kids."

When most customers walked in, they'd look at me as if I were an intruder, an invading female in this man's domain. But then Dewey would introduce Lee and me as husband and wife and give us some kind of compliment. The introduction made the point that my presence had Dewey's blessing. If the new-comer listened to Lee, it was obvious why I was there. Most new arrivals quickly forgot about me and started chatting with gusto. I guessed my presence didn't dampen the environment too much.

Once Lee's turn was announced and he was settled in the barber's chair, Dewey would prime a story, and Lee would jump on it with delight. Dewey probed for details, and Lee would gladly respond by weaving intricate tales about his life long ago, often with information I'd never heard. The guys sitting in the waiting chairs seemed enthralled.

Sadly, the trips to the shop became difficult over time. The multiple conversations in the cramped space started to stress Lee out, and he got grouchy with me.

"Let's drive by to see how many are waiting for Dewey's chair," I began to say to Lee on haircut day. "If there are more than one or two, we can go back later."

He liked that approach. To improve our chances, I asked Dewey which days and times tended to be slower. The effort was worth it. Lee absolutely relished the shop's storytelling and that he was treated like a regular guy while there. He always left Dewey's smiling and chatty. On the way out, I loved to tease Lee, saying that he was my suav-ey and de-bone-er husband, and he never failed to laugh heartily as I mispronounced those two words.

CAREGIVING LITE

I'd been dealing with spinal problems for years. By 2012, the tingling and numbness in my hands and arms were waking me off and on all night, every night. The annual MRI this year confirmed it was time to remove a disc and fuse the C4 through C7 vertebrae in my neck.

I made every preparation I could think of, including signing an "on hold" contract with a home-health agency so they could care for me in case the recovery was longer than expected. Lee's younger son and his family offered to care for him while I was in the hospital. Lee overheard conversations as I made plans and caught on about the upcoming surgery. He started following me around the house with a deep furrow in his brow.

"What's going to happen to me?" he'd ask over and over. "Who's going to be here while you're gone?"

Most dementia patients I knew had a "special person" from whom they drew confidence and a feeling of security, an advocate who instinctively understood their needs and desires and who would fight for them. Dementia patients typically wanted these special persons around as much as possible, especially when something unfamiliar was happening. During my hospital preparations, Lee surprisingly verbalized that he was uncomfortable with the idea that I wouldn't be with him and that I was risking a serious surgery. Thankfully, reassurances about my surgery and details from his family about their fun plans helped to reduce Lee's stress. I was determined to get it over with and had a sense that everything would work out fine.

The surgery went well, and Lee was brought to visit me in the hospital a couple of times. He smiled often and seemed carefree. I could tell he was having fun with his family. It was a huge relief that he was doing so well.

The recovery instructions required me to lie in an inclined bed at home for four weeks, to wear a neck brace at all times except when carefully showering, and to avoid lifting anything weighing more than a pound or two. A friend from church planned to spend a couple of hours each morning during the first week helping—washing dishes, doing laundry, and going to the store. It gave me a reassuring feeling to know that someone would be at the house with us, too. On my first full day at home, when Ruby offered to make Lee breakfast, he refused to touch it or even to be in the same room with her. She offered to take him out to lunch or for a ride, and Lee reacted with disgust at the prospect of being out with another woman. By the second day, Ruby felt so uncomfortable that she shortened her stay, and then she didn't return on the third day. I understood.

Lee paced around the house while I slept through most of the first day. The pain pills really knocked me out and made me feel as if I couldn't catch my breath. When I also broke out in a rash, the doctor stopped the hydrocodone pain medicine, certain I was allergic to it. He switched me to another pain medicine, but I just wasn't comfortable with being so drugged up during the day while Lee roamed aimlessly around the house. I decided to just take regular Tylenol instead. Then, two days later, I did the same during the night, out of fear that Lee would need help in the night and I wouldn't be able to hear him. That first week was awfully painful, but bearable.

During the first three or four days of the recovery, my daughter came by late afternoons to help me shower and to bring us prepared dinners. Lee reacted poorly to having her around and to the grandkids, too, even though they were familiar. My daughter cut their visits short. Lee just seemed so out of sorts. My fortitude plummeted; all I could do was cry. It was impossible for me to think clearly, what with the pain, fatigue, and aftermath of anesthesia. I had a sense that Lee and I were barely hanging on. In the midst of this low point, Lee walked into my bedroom with a ziplock baggie filled with ice, suggesting that I put it on my neck to help with the pain. I could see in his eyes that he was terrified and trying to do the best he could.

That little act of compassion settled my nerves, but even so, the first week post-surgery was the most difficult challenge I'd ever faced since Lee's diagnosis. Each day, it was all I could do to make sure that he took his medications and ate the breakfasts and lunches that I slapped together. I microwaved dinners that I had prepared and frozen weeks earlier and gingerly kept him company at the dining-room table while he ate. We managed to get through his bedtime and evening medication routines. I ran the dishwasher, ignoring the rest of the housework. In between these tasks, I lay in bed while Lee paced between his recliner and my bedroom. By the time we went to bed at night, we both felt beat up, completely spent. And I was in real pain.

Somehow, slowly, day by day, my determination and confidence started building back, partly because I knew this situation was temporary. By the fifth week post-surgery, I only needed to lie in bed for one hour three times a day, and while Lee resented my time in bed, he coped. My daughter and Lee's younger daughter-in-law took turns driving us to my physical-therapy appointments, which were twice a week for the first six weeks. Getting out of the house really perked up Lee's spirits. He relished people-watching and chatting in the lobby while waiting for my therapy sessions to be finished.

I wish I had taken videos of Lee the first couple of times we went out alone in our car during the seventh week post-surgery. He was beaming and looked so relieved to have his life back to normal. However, life wasn't yet normal for me. I couldn't scrub the bathrooms or vacuum the carpet or change the sheets or iron his shirts. To manage, I made use of a housekeeping service and a dry cleaners' laundry service for the shirts. Having two stranger housekeepers show up and work in the house really stressed Lee out, so I took him out for the two hours each week. I knew I was very fortunate to have this help during my recovery and often thought of those caregivers who didn't.

Within a few more weeks, my neck was doing well, and I was able to see the good that had come out of the surgery experience. The surgery and recovery had helped me to realize that the world wouldn't fall apart if I lowered my housekeeping standards or couldn't fulfill Lee's every wish. It also forced me to learn how to live with Lee's new crankiness without letting it affect my own state of mind. That ability to rise above his moods would serve me well later.

I also had one more important insight as a result of the surgery—that there is no middle ground when it comes to dementia caregiving. The role is full tilt or not; there is no half-way caregiving, no "caregiving lite." If ever, ever, ever I needed to recuperate at home again, I pledged to myself to make arrangements to have Lee stay elsewhere until I was ready to take over full-time caregiving.

Once ten weeks of recuperation were over, I went back to work part time and then transitioned to full-time work two weeks later. After having spent 24/7 with Lee for more than two months, I felt much less confident about leaving him alone each day and started looking into early retirement.

ARCHIVIST AND ADVOCATE

I am a person who likes to feel prepared. After spending so much time with Lee post-surgery, I worried: *What if there is an emergency while I am at work and Lee can't figure out how to get help?* I taped my cell and work numbers to our house phone and to the back of Lee's cell phone, hoping that would help. It was reassuring that Lee seemed able to reach me anytime he wanted. He would call me at work to ask how to use the remote for the TV, to ask where a picture album was, to ask when I was coming home, to tell me that the online bank account was frozen, or to say that he had just taken a shower. Thankfully, my manager understood.

While driving home from work one day, it dawned on me that I hadn't heard from Lee at all that afternoon. When I pulled into the garage, he also wasn't waiting at the back door to greet me as usual. I quickly found him in the living room, lying back in his recliner, slumped at an angle, sunken into the cushions, with a vacant look on his face.

"Lee?" I said, putting my hand on his shoulder. "Are you OK?"

"I feel sick," he answered faintly.

I felt his forehead—no fever. I had no idea what was going on but knew that he wasn't well. *Could it be his heart?*

"We're going to the hospital," I announced. His lack of protest scared me even more.

Lee sat very still in the chair next to me as I answered the ER receptionist's questions and gave the vague reason for the trip in—I knew something was very wrong but had no idea what because he had Alzheimer's disease and couldn't describe how he felt. She asked me for a quick summary of Lee's medical history, and once his past heart attacks came up, a staff member quickly took us to an examination room.

The emergency-room doctor walked into Lee's room right after the nurse had taken his vital signs.

"Do you have pain anywhere?" he asked.

"No," Lee said.

"Can you describe your symptoms?"

"I feel fine," Lee replied. "I don't know why my wife brought me in here."

I shouldn't have been shocked by that answer, but I was. The doctor looked frustrated and started walking toward the door. I panicked, thinking that he was giving up.

"He has Alzheimer's," I said.

"Yes, I know," the doctor curtly replied. I glanced at the nurse, who had a sympathetic expression on her face.

"Lee," I jumped in, "do you have a headache?"

"No."

The doctor shot me a dirty look; I was stepping into his business and knew immediately it was a mistake.

"Doctor," I said, "can I please speak with you out in the hall for a second?"

As I walked out of the room, the nurse took Lee's hand and chatted about the day's weather. Out in the hall, I explained to the doctor that during the last six months, Lee had never said he felt cold, even when he was shivering. He never claimed to be hungry or hot or to have pain. I had to look for clues and ask very specific questions, which sometimes elicited useful information but oftentimes didn't.

"Is there a way you can examine my husband and figure this out without his input?" I asked.

The doctor turned and, with an irritated look on his face, walked back into the exam room.

"I'm going to take a look at your eyes," he said, stepping up to Lee and turning on his little flashlight. "OK . . . good. Now, can you open your mouth for me?"

Immediately, the doctor took a step back. Lee's tongue and gums were nearly dry, with a whitish tinge. He was severely dehydrated, the doctor declared in a less stressed-out tone now that he had solved the mystery.

"You need to drink a big glass of water every afternoon from now on," he told Lee. "Today, I'm going to give you a big drink of water through an IV."

The two men laughed at the corny joke.

The doctor added, "As soon as you're done with the IV, you'll be able to go home, probably in an hour."

Lee gave the doctor a big smile and leaned back in the inclined bed, happy that he didn't have to stay long.

It was so hard to believe that with all of the phone calls he made every day for small things, Lee didn't think to call me when he felt deathly ill. Later that night, I came to grips with the fact that, while Lee was still able to figure out how to use the phone, he was no longer capable of recognizing emergencies. I sank into the fear of walking into the house after work to find him dead. All of these thoughts kept me tossing and turning in bed that night, well into the early-morning hours. *What if the ER doctor had not been willing to take the time needed to blindly investigate what was wrong?*

My caregiver friends and I had slowly transitioned to become our husbands' archivists, which meant we were now entrusted with the responsibility of tracking and reporting medical symptoms and health histories about illnesses, surgeries, vaccinations, and medications . . . all of the information our spouses never could have remembered. Lee was instinctively aware of my role and grabbed my attention immediately if he happened to have a clue that he was unwell. There was always an urgency in his voice at those times. I believe he knew that the physical awareness he sporadically felt was fleeting, like an apparition that crystallized, then evaporated.

And so, I kept track of changes doctors made to his medications and administered them at the appointed times. Physical therapists taught me prescribed exercises so I could make sure Lee did his homework exercises between appointments. I made doctors' appointments for follow-up visits for medical conditions that Lee forgot he had. The responsibility for Lee's health seemed so much heavier than when I was responsible for my children's health back in the day. Maybe it was because Lee was an adult who could at times convince naive medical providers that nothing was wrong. He could also fight me much more convincingly and pugnaciously about complying with doctors' orders than my children did when they were young.

There were many wonderful doctors who lightened my load, who understood the caregiver's archivist role and who were masterful communicators. They wove in a caregiver's input during an appointment without the patient ever noticing. Lee's neurologist was one of them. He always broke the ice with a discussion about our college football team. Once he turned the topic to Lee's health, the doctor would ask Lee a question and give him plenty of time to answer, then turn to me to ask if I agreed. Somehow, the doctor conveyed that he wasn't suggesting that Lee was wrong, but that people could have differences of opinion. Since Lee answered the doctor's question first, I had time to think about the most diplomatic way to offer "my opinion," if needed. Lee didn't seem offended by this approach.

In the later years of Lee's disease, I heard a suggestion to use notes. When Lee's symptoms worsened greatly, I stealthily slipped a note to the receptionist at check-in, while Lee was looking around for a seat. "This note is for the doctor to read before Lee's exam," an attached Post-it explained. That allowed me to get a quick bit of information about the dementia changes to the doctor without embarrassing or upsetting Lee. If I had it to do over again, I would have used this note communication method with all of his doctors anytime there were significant changes in any condition. Lee always left the neurologist's office with a smile.

The doctors who didn't seem to understand that patients with dementia weren't reliable sources of information only asked for my input very quickly at the end of an appointment or not at all. They often made me feel that any contribution I made was not welcome. I assumed this was due to time constraints. If important information was not mentioned at some point during an appointment or was told incorrectly, and if I suspected that information could affect a diagnosis or treatment, I waited for a pause to quickly slip it in. Sometimes this offended Lee and occasionally a doctor, who seemed to feel that I was unduly interjecting myself into the visit. I often left this type of appointment feeling embarrassed and mentally drained.

When I raised this physician-communication issue at a support-group dinner, the women exploded with pent-up frustrations. In fact, they vented for over an hour. All had dealt with multiple doctors who had made them feel like intruders at appointments. They all felt that they had to constantly prove their credibility—even though these same doctors knew they were taking care of their spouses day in and day out. The women shared that in order to offer important information, they had to communicate quickly and with a deferential demeanor. Even then, the physicians would somehow let them know their input was not appreciated.

In Lee's case, I would venture to estimate that a quarter of the physicians who had treated him since the dementia diagnosis didn't seem to understand the caregiver's archivist role. If I thought that I had information that would make a difference in a diagnosis or treatment plan, I pushed on to volunteer that information as concisely as possible, regardless of a physician's reaction.

Now that I knew Lee was unable to recognize an emergency, I no longer felt comfortable leaving him alone for more than a couple of hours. I submitted my paperwork to retire at the earliest possible date, on my sixty-second birthday. Lee was beyond ecstatic when I told him I was retiring in three months, on the first of February, 2013.

CHAPTER 3

2013

During 2013, the fatigue that is so common in those with dementia became more and more impactful on Lee. It seems to me now in hindsight that we both could sense the storm clouds on the horizon and scurried to fit in as many bucket-list adventures as we could.

WHILE WE STILL COULD

For some years before we met, Lee was a snowbird, living the winter months in a thirty-two-foot motor home that he drove down to Casa Grande, Arizona. He seemed drawn to Sedona and the Phoenix-Scottsdale areas. For my part, I had fallen in love with Arizona during a statewide vacation the year before we met. So, it was natural that, once I retired in February of 2013, we would take a celebratory trip to Phoenix.

Lee told everyone that he was looking forward to traveling, and he seemed genuinely excited to be going to Arizona. Yet I got the feeling that he was nervous about the flight. He'd never been anxious at all about past air travel and was a veteran of more than a hundred flights during his twenty-seven years in the Air Force. In fact, in his twenties, Lee had a temporary duty assignment as a member of an Air Force basketball team, flying back and forth from his detachment in Turkey to Africa for the team's basketball practices and to Germany for the games. When he could get more than one day of leave at a time, he grabbed space-available flights, often on Air Force hops, visiting Scandinavia, the Ethiopian bush, and most of the places in between. After he had coached me through flights in our early marriage until I understood that turbulence was not a threat, it seemed so unexpected that he was now anxious about flying.

I did everything that I could think of to try to make my retirement-celebration trip as easy as possible. I booked a flight that was nonstop, taking less than two hours. I kept his tickets, ID, and documents with me, so he didn't worry about losing them. I requested the seats with the extra four inches of legroom. I tucked snacks and an iPod loaded with movies into my carry-on backpack and bought canned drinks at the airport. At luggage check-in, I requested the free wheelchair service, which Lee balked at until he was cruising effortlessly down the long terminal hallways. I gave a running "time left before boarding" countdown to quell his fear about missing our flight. All of these preparations helped, but Lee still looked stressed throughout the trip.

A cold wind, socked-in skies, and rain greeted us as we stepped outside the Phoenix airport. Lee was extremely disappointed. His favorite thing to do, and perhaps the whole point of visiting Arizona in the winter, was to sit out on the hotel grounds and take in the sun. A homey breakfast restaurant, one that had good reviews and that was near our hotel, salvaged the vacation. The daily breakfasts were followed up by half-hour sightseeing drives into the Arizona desert, where the cactus just happened to be blooming. Each day, we toured one of Scottsdale's small specialty museums and ended these sightseeing excursions with lunches at little local spots on the way back to the hotel. By 1:00 p.m., Lee needed a three-hour nap; we followed that up with a stroll on the grounds for a few minutes before dressing for an early dinner. On our last day in Scottsdale, we finally saw the sunshine at brunch; Lee was in heaven! He fared remarkably well on that vacation and had completely forgotten about the bad weather by the time we arrived home.

I was really happy that Lee had enjoyed the trip, but for my part, the retirement-celebration trip was depressing. I had failed to adjust my expectations to realistically anticipate abrupt endings to outings, like museum visits, after just fifteen or twenty minutes or whenever Lee got fatigued and wanted to go to the car. I had not pictured spending hours every afternoon sitting in our hotel room while he slept. To be honest, it was disappointing to think that this was the retirement vacation I'd been anticipating for at least a decade. My husband was unable to think of my needs at all now, unlike our first years together. On that trip, I had to come to grips with the fact that our lives were entirely centered around Lee and his dementia now.

After returning home, I assumed Lee wouldn't want to travel anymore due to the recent anxiety about flying. So I was surprised when a couple of months later, Lee and his younger son began talking about a July trip to Iowa to take in some of Lee's favorite childhood places that he'd cherished while growing up and to visit with extended family and childhood friends. Lee's younger son and I agreed it was a now-or-never father-son trip.

Taking a flight just a couple of hours after Lee left town, I traveled to my hometown, too. Five days later, my return flights were booked for early in the day so I would arrive home before Lee. When I answered the front door and took one look at his face, I immediately thought, *This is the face of a man with one foot in the grave.* He could barely get himself over the threshold into the house.

"This trip was nearly too much for him," Lee's son explained. "Dad fought using a wheelchair at the airports."

There had been no nonstop flight options available to and from Omaha, so the trip home had included two flights. As luck would have it, those two flights connected at opposite ends of a Denver terminal. Lee literally fell onto the bed and slept the rest of that homecoming day and night. Once he recovered, though, both father and son said that the trip was definitely worth the effort. Lee expressed real gratitude as he looked through the pictures that his son had taken, saying they'd checked off everything on his wish list while there. Lee's yen to travel was satisfied. But I hadn't seen the maternal half of my extended family for at least a decade, and I was hoping to also visit them before the dementia got worse. Lee and his son were open to my taking a long-weekend trip, so I dashed off to Georgia. My visit with the Southern half of my extended family really lifted my spirits, and Lee had a great time with his college-age grandson, who stayed at our house while I was gone. Lee didn't seem at all disturbed by my absence. During July of 2013, each of us had been able to work our way through our most important bucket-list to-dos while we still could.

LIVING ON THE EDGE

Three or four days after I returned home from Georgia, I woke up with a start at 2:00 a.m. Something felt very wrong with my body, and there was a dark, foreboding sense in the pit of my stomach. Once I realized that I couldn't stand up to get out of bed, I crawled on all fours to the bathroom, then to where I kept my heart medication, taking a pill several hours early just in case it would help whatever was going on. Still, the feeling of doom got stronger and stronger. All at once, I just had to be with my husband, so I crawled down the hall to Lee's room and got myself up onto his bed. He immediately woke up.

"Can you please get my cell phone from the nightstand in my bedroom?" I asked with urgency in my voice.

While he did that, I called 911 from the landline phone on his nightstand.

"I think I'm having some kind of heart problem and need the paramedics," I told the dispatcher quickly, and then rattled off our address.

Lee handed my cell phone over and stood looking at me with terror on his face. Keeping the landline phone up to my right ear, I entered my passcode and raised the cell phone to my left ear to ask Siri to call Lee's younger son, who lived nearby. He answered right away despite the hour and quickly understood that I needed him to meet us at the hospital so that he could care for his dad. The call took less than a minute.

After hanging up the cell phone, I turned back to answer a few questions from the dispatcher while sounds from the other side of the house let me know that Lee had heard me quickly ask him to open the front door for the paramedics.

The room began to close in on me just as a paramedic suddenly appeared from out of my cloudy peripheral vision, stepping near the bed. I yanked off my Road ID medical bracelet, which listed my medications and health conditions, and handed it to him. When he started to ask me some questions, I interrupted.

"My husband has Alzheimer's," I said. "He can't be left alone. His son will pick him up at the hospital."

The paramedic nodded as a wave of nausea swept over me.

"Lee," I shouted. "Get me the bathroom trash can!"

He handed it to me just before I began to get sick. I leaned over the side of the bed and then immediately blacked out.

I had been unconscious for many hours and could barely

get my eyes open as I was being wheeled down a hall and into a cardiac intensive-care hospital room. Once I opened my eyes, they quickly squeezed shut again because the room was swimming. In those first few seconds they were open, though, I was able to catch a glimpse of sunlight coming into the room and some blurry figures sitting on chairs along the opposite wall. I remember being very confused, wondering who the people sitting in my room were, and thinking, *I'm way too tired for company.*

One of the visitors let me know that the spur-of-the-moment emergency arrangement for Lee had worked. The paramedics had understood the need to put him in the front passenger seat of the ambulance, and Lee's younger son had been waiting at the ER for him.

A nurse placed a damp washcloth over my eyes to help reduce the severity of the vertigo. Then I heard Lee's older son's voice asking me where my local daughter was, saying that he had been trying very hard to reach her. I couldn't remember where she was, that she and her family had gone to a remote area up north with spotty cell service. In fact, my brain felt as if it had short-circuited and was in a deep fog. Yet I was aware enough to feel relief to hear that someone was thinking for me, trying to reach my daughter for me.

After I'd been lying in bed with my eyes closed for a little while, I faintly heard some of the family talking with a nurse, and then a doctor, but couldn't make out what they were saying and didn't really have the energy to care. Now the shoe was on the other foot; I was the one needing an advocate. I relaxed as I heard Lee's two sons, his older daughter, and her husband step in to fill that role.

From the moment I regained consciousness, I experienced an overwhelming feeling that I had nearly died, and each visitor's tone of voice confirmed that. And I also had a deep-down sense that everything that could be done for me was being done. So, I settled back into bed, putting my fate in God's hands and saying a brief, silent prayer to thank Him for keeping me alive so far. Later that day, I learned that my heart rate had dropped to five beats per minute when being placed in the ambulance and that it was still at that rate when the ER doctor and on-call cardiologist first examined me. They still didn't know why.

"I've never had to show another doctor an ECG strip that was seven feet long before," the cardiologist joked that first day. To this day, I have no idea how the amazing paramedics and physicians kept me alive or how the on-call cardiologist in the ER got my heart rate back to normal. A doctor who came by my room one day did tell me it took hours to get my heart rate and blood pressure normalized.

Lee was eventually brought up for a visit on my first day in the hospital.

"Thank you," I softly said to my husband as I looked deep into his eyes, "for being by my side when I needed you most."

He smiled proudly but said little. A couple of days later, Lee was dropped off in my room by a family member so he and I could have a short visit. Another family member was scheduled to pick him up a half hour later. As soon as Lee and I were alone in my room, he declared that he had to go to the restroom and left. I overheard a nurse in the hall giving him directions to the public restroom and could hear it wasn't close. The hospital was huge, with multiple wings and floors. When he didn't return after a while, I pushed my call button.

"My husband has Alzheimer's and went to the restroom somewhere. I'm not sure he can find his way back," I told the nurse, and she immediately ran off to look for him.

Lee was eventually found wandering the halls, lost. The family member who had brought him for the visit and I realized that Lee couldn't be left alone with me even for a few minutes while I was immobile, hooked up to monitors as I lay in bed.

I was in cardiac intensive care for five days and then in the telemetry department for another quick hospital stay three weeks later after I had a pacemaker implanted. Lee did remarkably well. After overseeing his care during their trip the month before, Lee's younger son knew his medication schedule and other needs. Lee seemed to take my middle-of-the-night illness and my absences in stride, then quickly forgot about them. After I was discharged, my cardiologist encouraged me to ease into walking or exercise, but I never found a way to make that happen.

ONE MORE LAST TRIP

Lee and I went to one or two away games every season to support our local college football team. We had even made the fan pilgrimage to the epic 2007 Fiesta Bowl, where our team beat Oklahoma 43 to 42 in a nail-biter in overtime—making the Statue of Liberty play and the "football-game marriage proposal" watercooler topics that season. The 2010 Fiesta Bowl wasn't as gripping, but that win was extremely satisfying in its own way. Dressed in full fan regalia as we passed through the Biltmore Hotel bar on the way to our room, we grinned like Cheshire cats as the TCU fans gritted their teeth and congratulated us on our team's 17-to-10 win.

By 2013, after our disappointing February "retirement trip" to Phoenix and his challenging July trip to Iowa, I was sure that Lee's traveling days were over. But news about the team was bubbling up in early August on the local TV and radio stations, and the coverage was getting Lee excited for the coming season. Just a week or two after I had received my pacemaker,

Lee lobbied hard to take a trip to the big season opener in Seattle, against the University of Washington. Seattle was only an hour's flight away. The booster club had contracted with a travel agency to charter an inexpensive flight on the day before the game and to arrange a charter bus to take fans from Sea-Tac airport directly to a very nice downtown hotel with discounted rooms. The bus would also shuttle boosters to and from the game on Saturday and then back to the airport on Sunday. These arrangements made the trip as laid-back as possible. I couldn't say no.

After the flight and the bus trip to the hotel, Lee was exhausted but not sick-tired. He watched TV and dozed in bed all afternoon, had a relaxing dinner at the hotel restaurant, and slept unusually well that night. This was going better than I'd expected. The next morning, we were raring to go. A couple of hours before we were to meet the bus outside the hotel entrance for the ride to the stadium, we walked to the Starbucks around the corner to get egg-and-ham sandwiches for breakfast. While waiting inside the tiny, crowded coffee shop for our order, Lee started slurring his speech. Then he tried multiple times to hand a twenty-dollar bill to the cashier, even though he'd already paid. I got a sinking feeling after I noticed that his eyes were drooping and that he was walking cattywampus, like a drunk. *Is Lee having a stroke?* I got the sandwiches to go and quickly herded him back up to our room. On the phone, Lee's younger son told me to check his dad's medications. Had he taken extra by accident? Yes, he had! In fact, I discovered that Lee had taken *all* of that day's daytime *and* nighttime pills, all at once, first thing that morning.

"If it's just one day's medications, then it won't kill him," his son reassured me. "He'll need to sleep it off but should be normal by your flight tomorrow."

I hung up the phone and took a deep breath.

"Lee," I said, pasting a smile on my face. "You accidentally took too many pills. You need to go to bed."

Lee stiffened his spine. "Hell no," he boomed at me. "I'll take a short nap, but I am *not* missing the game."

"OK, all right," I said, relieved that he'd agreed to a nap and expecting that, once he dozed off, he'd be down for hours. *I hope he won't be mad at me when he wakes up,* I thought, trying to assuage my own disappointment about missing the game.

After eating his sandwich and then sleeping for an hour, Lee woke himself up with a start and announced that he was going downstairs to wait for the bus, then pushed past me to the hotel-room door. I grabbed our sweatshirts and my purse and, while making sure the hotel-room key card and tickets were inside, ran to catch up. He still looked drunk, but there was no stopping him!

We arrived at the gathering spot outside the hotel entrance just in time to make the charter bus. Some of our fellow boosters stared at Lee, who staggered as we approached. I leaned in toward them and whispered, "He mistakenly took his nighttime pills."

They smiled, nodded, and helped to get him on and off the bus, making his impaired state seem all in good fun. Lee laughed the whole time—he thought those boosters were a riot as they teased him! At the stadium, we managed to make it on our own to our nearby seats in the disabled section, and his wooziness lessened as the morning wore on. By kickoff, Lee had willed himself to nearly full alertness. I could tell that he was functioning on pure adrenaline, so excited to be at the season opener.

After the game, Lee collapsed onto the hotel bed and slept until the next morning, feeling great by the time the bus pulled up for the ride to the airport. It was definitely a memorable game. This really did end up being our last trip, once and for all.

TRADITION

Lee still expected to attend home football games, since doing so had been our tradition for at least fifteen years. I strategized every possible way to get him to the first home game of this season. At the same time, I was a little amazed at the irony of the situation, that I was working so hard to attend a football game.

One of the first questions I'd asked when we met was whether Lee was a sports fan and, specifically, whether he was into football. With wide-open, innocent-looking eyes, he had sworn all those years ago that he had no interest *at all* in sports. (He admitted three years later that he could tell I was looking for a "no" answer.) During our first year, I never saw him watch a game on TV or even appear remotely interested in sports. I was convinced and relieved.

The truth came out, drip by drip, during our second year together, as he chatted with his older son in earnest about the local college team's quarterback. Lee dropped interesting factoids on me about this player's high-school career or that player's hometown and family, knowing such information would endear these players to me. Eventually, he talked me into going to a home game.

"The weather's so beautiful," he said, as sweet as pie. "Wouldn't it be fun to sit outside in the sun, at the stadium?"

I reluctantly agreed. "I'll go just this once, to support my alma mater."

At our very first game, Lee explained what was happening in a way that was entertaining and accessible. It was impossible not to get excited when the team made a first down, what with the entire stadium on their feet, shouting and waving their arms in the air. Over that first season, I learned to recognize when a player made a face mask or holding penalty, and I came to love those long arching passes during which the crowd held its collective breath. I couldn't help but jump up and down when the defense stopped a promising play or kept an opponent from earning an extra point. I was proud to yell out, "And that's another Bronco first down!" and knew when it was the right time to give forth with the cheer. Lee jumped up for the good plays and high-fived our seatmates after the great plays. By the end of that year, I had my own blue-and-orange team sweatshirt, and we had season tickets for the 1998 and '99 season. Eventually, we got a parking place at the stadium for the motor home and hosted family tailgate parties for a few years.

In recent years, I had paid the optional fee for a space in the parking garage and made sure we arrived early enough to get one of its disabled spaces. But by 2013, the half-mile walk to the stadium was impossible for Lee. That year I learned that the university offered a disabled riders' shuttle bus between the garage and the stadium and that it ran every ten minutes. *This'll be easy*, I thought.

As soon as the bus doors swung open, I gulped. That first step was nearly knee-high, well beyond Lee's reach with his inflexible hips and legs. And the stairs were far too narrow for me to fit in next to Lee so I could help to lift him up.

If this bus is for the disabled, then why isn't there some kind of help for people who can't manage these stairs? I thought to myself. Because Lee wasn't in a wheelchair, the lift was out.

"We can do this!" I said to my husband in a voice that conveyed a confidence I didn't feel. I stood behind him and firmly supported his back as he leaned back to slowly raise his right foot, inch by inch, up toward that first step. Once he finally got the tip of his right shoe resting on the edge of the stair, he leaned forward to grab the railing and pulled hard on it while I pushed him up from behind. At one point in the process, Lee was completely leaning back on me, which I knew was dangerous. Eventually, he was able to get his other foot solidly on the step. The whole process was exhausting and embarrassing, especially when I looked up and saw the bus driver scowling at us. After we were seated on the bus, I patted Lee on the back, cheering him on and silently thinking about the return trip.

The bus went directly to the entrance of the stadium marked for those with disabilities. As we walked in, I encouraged Lee to make a pit stop on the way to our seats. (It was nearly impossible to get him all the way back to the restroom once a game started.) Our seats were on the forty-yard line, in the fifth row, which is nine stairsteps up from ground level. The stairs didn't have a railing, but I'd done research on helping Lee up the stairs. My physical therapist told me to grab hold of the back of Lee's belt and to use it like a gait belt, standing at his side to pull him as he stepped up, then to steady him on each step.

"Ask someone to stand in front of Lee, on the next step up," the PT advised, "so he can hold on to the person's shoulders or waist or belt for balance."

Thank goodness for the kindness of strangers. A big guy who had a seat near ours positioned himself at Lee's right and held him under his right arm, lifting him with each step. I was on Lee's left. Another fan stood behind to support Lee if he started to lean back. He hated all the hubbub, but I think he knew he needed the help. By the time we reached Lee's seat on the aisle, he was winded but still excited to be at the game. I relaxed into my seat, feeling grateful for our stadium neighbors and somewhat shocked at how difficult it was just getting Lee to a game this year.

The sky was as clear and blue as could be, a perfect day for this season opener. Yet I could tell that the loud beat of

the music that played during the teams' warm-ups was difficult for Lee. With each minute that passed, the furrows on his
brow got deeper. After several grouchy comments, the music
blessedly stopped. Lee got to his feet (along with the entire stadium) for the kickoff, and then watched the game with happy
concentration, commenting on every play and cheering on the
team.

After the game, we waited in the shuttle line at the front
of the stadium for nearly half an hour, joined by at least a hundred others jostling for position. When the bus pulled up,
younger people who were not obviously disabled pushed past
us; Lee was terrified. I reverted to the more assertive practices
of my city upbringing, shielding Lee and trying to hold our
place in line. Quite a few did force their way past us, but we
made it onto the second bus that came along. I know Lee heard
the catty remarks from those behind us about how slowly he
climbed the stairs while I pushed from behind. By the time we
got to our car, I was pissed off, plain and simple, and Lee was
thoroughly spent.

*Why isn't there some kind of oversight for the boarding pro-
cess for a disabled riders' bus? Why can't people who need the
lift use it, maybe with a bus's spare wheelchair? Why is the public so impatient with those who are obviously disabled?* I ranted
on silently to myself.

Lee was sick-tired by the time we got home. He ended
up going to only one more game during the 2013 season. It
looked like this tradition was going to join the list of impossible pleasures.

A SHRINKING DOMAIN

Throughout our courtship and early marriage, Lee and I rode
bikes and took long walks along the twenty-five-mile greenbelt

that winds through our city, bordering the river. The path allowed us to view the river up close and, during the summer, to watch families and groups jubilantly tubing down it. In quieter sections of the river, we could see men standing in waders, casting long fishing lines to snag rainbow trout, brown trout, whitefish, and an occasional catfish. Lee had originally been drawn to settle here once he retired because of the easy access to great fishing all over the state. He still had his fly-tying equipment, rods, and reels and loved watching the water flow by.

As we walked along the greenbelt in the fall of 2013, bikers, runners, and other walkers said friendly hellos as they cautiously passed us by. Because we would be walking farther than Lee was able, I'd brought along a wheelchair. Lee pushed it in front of him, using it for support. When he got tired, he sat, and I pushed until he was ready to walk again. This was the first time we'd been on the greenbelt all year, and by the time we made it back to the car, he was pretty tired. It turned out that this walk would be the last time Lee would be able to visit this beloved place.

Lee also hadn't been able to go shopping for several years. He couldn't walk the distance from the car into the store, up and down the aisles, and then back out to the car. I had requested a disabled placard from Lee's primary-care physician, and he'd made the referral that same day to the DMV. Even with parking in the disabled spaces, the walking was still too much. So, I made brief shopping trips almost daily, in fifteen minutes or less, while Lee waited in the car. Yet it seemed such a shame that he never had the chance to peruse store shelves and select things on his own. In 2013, when I saw a motorized cart sitting near where we'd parked, I wondered what Lee's reaction would be if I steered it to the passenger side of the car. He had balked at using one during previous attempts in prior years. This time, he took the hint, got out of the car, and put one foot on the side edge of the cart while grabbing the steering wheel and attempting to pull himself up and onto the seat. But in order to sit on the cart, he had to squat and suspend his rear end as he slid under the steering wheel. He definitely did not have the thigh and rear-end muscle tone needed to do squats. On this first try, Lee lost his balance. I quickly pushed his back toward the seat as he pulled hard on the steering wheel. He managed to fall so his rear end hung onto the edge of the seat. It felt like that first attempt at using a cart was dangerous for the both of us.

Why doesn't the steering wheel swivel up or somehow get out of the way, so disabled riders can just sit down without having to squat, balance, and scoot? I wondered.

The controls were unmarked; we had to use trial and error to figure out how to operate the cart. Once in the store, Lee couldn't remember how the levers worked, so I showed him every few minutes. One time, while concentrating very hard on operating the cart, he accidentally knocked over a display case. In humiliation, he immediately steered straight for the door. I decided to keep trying on subsequent shopping trips, but available carts were few and far between. The handful of times Lee badly wanted to go into our nearest warehouse store, I went on the hunt, walking up and down the parking-lot rows and store aisles searching for an available cart. I never could find one that was unoccupied or not in the process of being charged. At one visit, I even stopped by the customer-service desk to see if the rep knew where any carts might be. He advised me that I should just push Lee around in his own wheelchair.

How can I push a shopping cart and my husband's wheelchair at the same time? I thought to myself. After a month of trying, Lee and I gave up on his going into stores.

By the fall of 2013, travel, football games, fishing, walks along the greenbelt, and shopping were all too difficult. Lee's domain was shrinking.

CHAPTER 4

2014

In the first two years after the diagnosis, 2009 and 2010, there was little obvious loss in Lee's thinking ability. During the next couple of years, the loss was noticeable to me, but Lee was still able to find ways to hide his deficits from those who didn't see him often or for more than a couple of hours. By the fifth year, 2014, it felt as if the cognitive and physical downturns picked up speed. It was no longer a surprise to anyone that Lee had Alzheimer's disease.

LOSING COGNITIVE GROUND

Near the end of 2013, the neurologist increased one of Lee's Alzheimer's medications up to its standard dose, now that Lee's nightmares were completely gone. After a few days, I began to see a remarkable improvement in Lee's awareness. He objected to not being able to drive. He protested when I paid the bills. He noticed and complained when he lost his debit card. He whined about having to take his medications. He tried to log on to our online bank account. He asked to see our monthly bank statements. He tried to turn on his favorite TV shows. He attempted to call family members on his flip cell phone. Before the medication increase, Lee had been oblivious to the fact that I handled so many tasks for him. After the medication increase, he became acutely aware of his cognition losses and was paranoid when he couldn't do a task, as if someone had sabotaged it. As a result, Lee often refused to talk with me and stormed off to bed.

Within a few months, though, Lee's awareness declined back to where it had been before the medication change. He returned to being oblivious about his deficits and was much less frustrated. Then he gradually declined even further.

Lee's mind became like a blackboard, with each day's events wiped clean every few hours or even every few minutes. However, one or two random facts or experiences did seem to hang on for a while. He might remember the name of a man he met in passing, or some bit of news about one of the grandchildren, or that he had spoken with an out-of-town friend recently. I thought that Lee must have been aware that he was losing some of his mental capacity. Lee's anxiety increased. If he happened to remember that he had plans—for example, to go to breakfast or lunch with a friend or family member—he would wake himself up at 4:00 a.m., worried about missing the outing despite the fact that he'd never missed any engagement. After a while, he even started keeping himself awake most of the night if he remembered he had plans, regardless of the day it was scheduled. So, I stopped giving Lee advance notice.

Movies and books were too difficult to follow now that his memory couldn't hold on to their plotlines. Instead, Lee watched cable news, sports, and weather, with their series of two-minute clips, each short enough for him to follow along. Classic Westerns were his favorites, with each scene or shootout now a separate story on its own.

Lee did still have long-term memories and often told

stories about his childhood and young adulthood. Many of these stories began to have triggers. When he saw or heard a trigger, it launched a corresponding, predetermined story, repeated almost word for word each time. For example, *every single time* he saw geese, he told me the exact same two stories, almost word for word—about why geese honk loudly as they fly in a V formation and why our local geese no longer migrated south. Lee had a bank of maybe fifty of these triggered stories. Our clergyman and physical therapist loved retelling me Lee's stories, which they had heard multiple times. They seemed to have a great affection for these stories and were amazed at how identical Lee's telling was each time he repeated one.

On scattered days, Lee anxiously asked questions over and over from the moment we left the house. "Where are we going?" he'd say, peering out the car window. "What time is it? What day is it?" And so on. I think Lee knew he was lost without my help.

Logic or any kind of multistep process was over Lee's head. For example, no matter how hard he tried, he could no longer figure out how to pump gas. Yet he didn't want me "sticking my nose into his business," so I sat in the car and waited for the inevitable. Lee would make multiple unsuccessful tries to pump the gas, and that made him paranoid and furious. I wondered, *Does his memory of working at his dad's gas station, pumping gas as a teenager, long before card scanners were used, confuse him?* On some occasions, Lee would realize he needed to pay at the pump first before lifting the nozzle. I'd sit in the car and watch in the side-view mirror while he tried working through the process. After five minutes of working through the steps in any order—searching for the debit card, fumbling with inserting the card into various spots on the pump, touching various buttons on the pump's screen, entering various PINs, putting the nozzle in and out of the fuel tank pipe—Lee would get exasperated. If people in line behind us began to get out of their cars to try to get a look at the cause of the holdup, I'd jump out, get the pump started, then jump back into the car, leaving Lee to finish up. Inserting myself into the process frustrated him to no end. He would become furious and refuse to talk with me for the rest of the day. Any process-driven task was a no-win situation for the both of us.

Even familiar cognitive processes he had completed daily were becoming too much. At the beginning of 2013, Lee solved the crossword puzzle in an hour every morning, as he had for decades. By 2014, he might read a clue and come up with the answer but not remember how to enter the letters in the appropriate boxes. At other times, he couldn't understand what a clue meant, almost as if it were in a foreign language. If he struggled, I'd give him the clue's definition or an obvious synonym for the answer, and he nearly always came up with the correct answer. Then I'd write the word in for him. He loved doing the puzzle this way, "as a team."

Lee's face would turn tomato red when he tried to use the cable-TV remote, often accidentally turning off the cable box or switching the input from cable to DVD. Eventually, I found a universal remote called the Flipper that was designed specifically for dementia patients. That inexpensive, very simple, and yet amazingly effective remote gave him back a little sense of control.

For decades, Lee had used university and government internet sites to create flight forecasts and weather forecasts for locations around the world. In years past, he would let me know if I could expect turbulence or any other weather-related effect on a flight. He competed against local TV meteorologists' forecasts, flawlessly predicting the local weather in greater detail and further out, almost as if he were showing off to me. Now, I navigated to the sites for Lee, but he couldn't remember which data to use or how to analyze it. Lee spent all of 2013 in frustration before finally giving up on weather forecasting for the family.

In late July, after seeing a couple of short clips about the 2007 Fiesta Bowl on the sports news, Lee said that he would like to watch that game again. We knew the game by heart, having viewed our DVD at least ten times in the past. I set up the DVD again that day, and as the game moved into the second quarter, Lee got more and more thrilled by every play, yelling and punching into the air in excitement. It took me a while to realize that he now thought the recorded game was live. His long-term memory of seeing the game in Phoenix was gone.

Lee became much less talkative in group conversations, perhaps guarding against revealing that he didn't remember much from the recent past. When Lee did converse with others, he reminisced about the distant past or focused on that odd story, current event, or fact that had randomly stuck from yesterday's news, weather, or sports TV show.

Lee was becoming very anxious to have me nearby at all times. My friends who had husbands at about the same stage of dementia said that their spouses were also becoming "clingy" to some degree. By this point, I couldn't leave a room without Lee calling me back after five minutes apart. That neediness made me think that he might know he was incapable of taking care of many situations that came up. By this point, I suspected that Lee knew he was losing cognitive ground.

DECLINES

Dementia is a category of diseases and conditions that typically cause a gradual degradation of a person's brain and overall physical condition. The decline is usually slow, taking place over many years, in many cases for a decade or more. However, I learned from experience that dementia's progression isn't always gradual.

Many of the people I knew with dementia experienced a steep decline—a drop in the condition of their health or ability to perform essential life functions—right after an illness or surgery. It seemed as if the person's body just couldn't withstand the dementia plus another health issue at the same time. These dementia declines came out of the blue, suddenly and for seemingly no reason at all. Some declines were minor, and others were significant. Some would reverse on their own, with the person improving days later just as suddenly as he had declined. Most of my support-group members' husbands had each experienced two or more dementia declines by the time they passed away. In 2014, medical researchers were trying to figure out why these sudden dementia declines happened.

Lee came down with a cold and an eye infection in early April 2014. Although his eyes recovered quickly with the help of an optical antibiotic cream, his overall condition declined. He became so exhausted that he could barely shave. Lee was able to walk independently in the morning but then became weaker as the day wore on. On bad days, he couldn't get up from a chair without help and would inhale deeply when he walked, as if he were steeling himself for a long journey. His appetite also dropped dramatically; he'd eat breakfast but then almost nothing else for the rest of the day. I tried everything I could think of to encourage Lee to eat so he wouldn't lose weight.

As I passed by Lee's recliner one day in April, I noticed that he was having what appeared to be a seizure. The minute areas all over his body spasmed independently of each other, nothing at all like the rhythmic jerking of epilepsy. This irregular twitching all over his body lasted about thirty seconds, which seemed like an eternity to me. Lee had been dozing before the seizure began and continued to sleep without noticing. I took him to his neurologist, and nothing unusual was found. The doctor said that a seizure might or might not happen again and was not unusual in Alzheimer's patients. I had seen small twitches in the muscles between Lee's thumb and pointer finger for years and had been told these were common among people with dementia or Parkinson's disease. But this whole-body involvement was something else entirely. A few years later, a friend's husband with Alzheimer's disease had such extreme seizures near the end of his life that he had to be placed on anti-seizure medication.

After a few weeks, Lee's appetite and strength improved, and the seizures never returned. The eye-infection-and-cold decline had completely reversed itself. I held my breath every day.

ACCOMMODATIONS

At the end of April, Lee said his left-hip pain was so bad that he needed to see a doctor. He had never asked to see a doctor before, so I knew the pain must be intense. By the day of the orthopedic surgeon's appointment, Lee could barely walk from the waiting room to the examination room. He leaned so heavily on me that I nearly toppled over. The nurse grabbed an office walker and shoved it in front of him.

During the exam, the surgeon moved Lee's leg into different positions. The doctor found that the hip joint rotated around just fine. Lee realized his hip was not painful; the pain was isolated in his back instead. An in-office X-ray of the hip was ordered just to be safe, and it confirmed that the joint was fine. On the way out, the nurse told us that a radiologist would read the X-ray as well. The next day, a radiology center called asking me to select an MRI appointment for Lee. I told the woman I'd call back, hung up the phone, and broke down in tears.

The memory of an MRI a year before came flooding back. When I'd made that radiology appointment a year ago, I'd explained to the scheduler, "MRIs are terrifying for my husband, so I'd like to go back to help get him dressed and to keep him calm. Would that be OK for this appointment?"

"No problem," the receptionist agreed.

But once we'd arrived at that appointment last year, the receptionist on duty wouldn't let me accompany Lee. I tried quickly and quietly to explain the need, but she didn't seem to care. Lee looked very concerned and glanced back at me as he was escorted through a door. As soon as he was out of sight, I went to another receptionist's window and told her that my husband had Alzheimer's and would freak out without me. This receptionist nodded and went to get a supervisor. In a minute, the supervisor appeared at the side door and took me right back.

As I walked the long hall that led back to the rooms with the radiology machines, I could hear Lee loudly arguing with someone about changing into a gown. I now understood why the supervisor had quickly brought me back without saying a word.

"There is no way I'm going to lie down on one of those tables!" Lee shouted.

Before we'd left home, I'd given Lee a light dose of an antianxiety medication prescribed by his family-practice physician for radiology appointments. It didn't help that day. *There is a fifty-fifty chance he is going to storm out of here,* I thought to myself. Somehow, I was able to divert his attention. After he changed into a gown, we stored his clothing in a locker and took the key, and the radiology tech and I were able to convince Lee to lie down on the machine's table for the MRI procedure.

After the MRI, Lee looked as if he'd been through a war.

I couldn't imagine what it was like for him, lying there in that claustrophobic metal tube with the incessant metal clanging inches from his head, especially when simple background music in restaurants made him want to jump out of his skin. Lee was traumatized, and my heart broke for him. It took days for him to recover. On that day, I promised Lee that I would never take him for another MRI.

Yet here we were a year later. I had explained to the orthopedic surgeon and the nurse at the beginning of last week's appointment about Lee's difficulty with last year's MRI. I wondered, *What could I have done differently to help them understand the situation?*

I never returned the call to the radiology center. A few days later, they called again, asking to make the appointment for the MRI. Feeling defeated, I complied. When the appointment day came and it was time to leave, Lee refused loudly. It seemed as if he remembered the traumatic experience from a year ago. I stood in the living room for a minute, weighing the options, then picked up the phone and canceled the appointment. *The X-ray showed that his hip joint was normal,* I thought. *The exam didn't indicate a problem either. Isn't that enough for someone in Lee's condition? I made my husband a promise a year ago, and I'm not going back on it.*

Two weeks later, the orthopedic office's receptionist called, asking why Lee hadn't had the MRI. I explained, and the receptionist said she would pass the information to the nurse.

Another two weeks later, the orthopedic office's nurse called and asked why Lee hadn't had the MRI; I re-explained.

One week after that, the office called again, this time asking to speak directly to Lee. I handed the phone off to him. When the receptionist asked Lee why he hadn't had the MRI, he said he didn't know anything about an MRI and abruptly hung up on her.

A few days later, a doctor called. I tried to explain but

couldn't find a way to help him grasp the magnitude of Lee's anxiety and difficulties with MRIs. Without any other way to communicate, I told him that if there was someone who wanted to take Lee to the MRI, I was fine with that, but that I just couldn't participate in re-traumatizing my husband. He backed off.

Finally, the radiology clinic called again. This time they asked to make an appointment for a CAT scan. *Thank goodness!*

When it came time, I was allowed to go back to help Lee through the appointment, and it was very fast and easy. In the end, there was nothing wrong with Lee's hip. He was never prescribed another MRI.

My caregiver friends had their own stories about having to go to bat for their spouses. They often talked about how difficult it was for them to communicate with medical professionals about the need for special accommodations during procedures that are far from routine for people with dementia.

THE "WIDOW-MAKER"

I adore babies but couldn't help but dread a baby shower on May 3, 2014. As the date approached, I kept having a deep-down, foreboding feeling that something was seriously wrong with Lee, something that we hadn't yet put our finger on. Leaving him alone for the entire afternoon made me feel very uncomfortable, especially since he no longer knew how to use the phone to call for help and since the party was on the east edge of town, at least a thirty-minute drive from home. I couldn't skip the shower without hurting the feelings of family members, yet I couldn't bear to stay for more than an hour. After I made it home to Lee and saw that he was fine, I felt silly for worrying.

Three days later, from my seat in the physical therapist's

waiting area, I could see Lee riding a stationary bike on the other side of a large room stocked with exercise equipment, tables, and mats. It seemed to me that he was pushing himself hard, too hard, but Jim, our physical therapist, seemed unperturbed. He and Lee were chatting away as the pedals went slowly around. I thought, *I must be mistaken about how hard Lee is working.*

Once finished, Lee trudged out to the waiting area, then told me that he was really, really tired. He seemed to be struggling to simply walk as we made it to the exit. Then Lee held tighter to my arm for support, with the expression of someone laboring to hike up a steep mountain trail as we made it the remaining fifteen feet from the office door to the building's elevator. Once he was settled in the car, Lee seemed to recover quickly and looked comfortable. I relaxed a little.

As we traveled west along a five-lane arterial roadway busy with noon traffic, Lee happily chatted about his conversation with the therapist. While driving, I spotted out of the corner of my eye a glimpse of his right hand being placed over his heart for about five seconds. He never did that. Immediately, I flashed back to the story I'd heard in my support group about a lady with dementia who'd made that very same hand movement, and it ended up being a sign of an impending heart attack. *Is this a red flag?* I wondered. *Should I take a left at the next light and rush the seven or so blocks to the ER? What if the hand movement is nothing? I would hate to put Lee through an exhausting visit to the ER.*

"Do you have any pain?" I asked. "Does your upper arm hurt?"

He replied no, with a serious look on his face.

Pulling up into our driveway ten minutes later, I finally thought to ask if there was anything unusual about how his chest felt and held my hand up in front of his heart without touching him.

"It feels like someone is pushing in real hard on my chest, right there," Lee said as he motioned over his heart. Panic washed over me.

As the paramedics pushed the gurney toward the ER door, I walked close behind. The ECG had indicated that a severe heart attack was imminent. At the same time, Lee kept saying that he felt fine and wanted to go to lunch. After he was moved into a room in the ER, family members rotated in, two at a time, and their visits kept him distracted. Lee was in the queue for the cath lab. A few hours later, we moved to a room on the cardiac floor to wait his turn.

Lee was tired but rested patiently as the hours ticked by. That night, the cardiologist's nurse practitioner came by and told me that if it got too late, or if the cardiologist felt too tired to do the procedure after his many hours in the cath lab, it might have to wait until tomorrow morning. At 2:00 a.m., Lee was finally taken away, and an hour later, the nurse practitioner came by to update family members and me as we sat in the surgery waiting area.

"You know, you saved your husband's life by taking it seriously when he put his hand over his heart. He was building up to a 'widow-maker' heart attack, but we caught it before the attack actually happened," she informed me.

Two new stents reopened the left anterior descending artery, which had been 96 percent blocked, and a couple more stents were also inserted where there were other blockages, too.

I'd known Lee's cardiologist for fifteen years. After the procedure, the doctor visited with me and carefully confided that there was nothing more that could be done for Lee's heart. I knew that Lee's chest had large staples holding the center of his sternum together, evidence of a past quadruple bypass done in the early 1990s. Lee joked about being a member of the "zipper club," but I suspected that those staples were nothing like a zipper, that they couldn't be reopened. And he'd had a couple of earlier stent procedures over the years. This time would be his last, the doctor said. Despite the doctor's troubling news, I was grateful that Lee had beaten the dire widowmaker's odds. He would just need to remain in the hospital for a couple of days to recover.

Lee was sedated, so I slipped out for a nap and a shower. By the time I returned, at 9:00 a.m., the drugs had worn off, and he was wide awake and upset.

"Honey, I'm right here," I said, sitting beside the bed and taking his hand. "I'm not going to leave again until you get discharged, I promise. I will be holding your hand all day and all night."

Lee seemed to sense that I meant it and settled down, especially that evening when he saw me lie down on a cot in his room and a nurse bring me a blanket. With all of the nurses' nighttime checks on Lee, I didn't sleep at all, and I recognized my body couldn't take another night in the hospital by Lee's side. Thankfully, he was discharged the next day.

I had hoped that, with the largest artery now open and more oxygen flowing to his heart, Lee would feel better and have more energy. Unfortunately, after he had settled back into his normal routine, he told me that he never felt well; he just made it through the day. Now I knew for certain that the fatigue was caused by the Alzheimer's disease.

CHANGING PERSONALITY

In 2014, Lee began to lose lifelong aspects of his personality. For example, activities that he previously loved to do, some as simple as sitting in the sun in our backyard or at a park, didn't interest him at all anymore. Lee had always been crazy about dogs. We'd had an Airedale for thirteen years, and he was crushed when Lucy passed away in 2013. In 2014, an adorable

Coton puppy became available, and the breeder offered to let me bring her home on a trial basis. She was a little white fluff-ball, the type of dog Lee had fawned over before. But now, he demanded that I immediately take her out of the house. Lee turned down neighbors' offers to pet their friendly dogs, too, something he'd always loved to do. It felt like I was losing my husband bit by bit.

Lee's stature and walk completely changed. And, for some unknown reason, he began to walk with his hands in his pockets, dangerous for an already unsteady person. I was fearful that he'd do a face-plant if he tripped. But when I begged Lee to take his hands out of his pockets, he would "pshaw" me, acting like he'd always walked that way.

Lee's incredible sense of direction was going. He had always instinctively known which way was north, east, south, and west, even when in the middle of an unfamiliar city with tall buildings blocking the horizon. He would nonchalantly find his way to any point in the United States and around colossal international cities without the use of any navigation aids. So, I was shocked when, on the way home from taking a ride in a familiar, rural part of the county, he kept asking where we were. He was lost and a little panicked. A month later, as we passed an intersection that we'd traveled through a hundred times before, Lee said he didn't recognize anything there. I could tell that the disorientation was freaking him out, so I started identifying cross streets as we passed them and giving him advance notice of landmarks. He still looked perplexed and anxious. On days when Lee was especially disoriented, I cut our rides short.

I could see that the Alzheimer's disease was gaining steam and beginning to eradicate his true personality. I think Lee sensed it, too. He often hugged me and told me he loved and appreciated me. I did what I could to reassure my husband.

ONE LAST TIME

In August 2014, Lee was pumped up for the first home game, having forgotten the difficulties of getting to and from the game a year ago. We parked in the same disabled parking area in the garage but didn't take the shuttle bus this time. Instead, I pulled out the lightweight travel wheelchair from the back of the car. Lee scowled at first, but once we got into the thick of tailgaters, cookouts, and the marching band's parade, he caught football-fan fever. Nothing but smiles at that point!

Pushing the wheelchair down the sidewalk along University Drive was more strenuous than I had expected, especially when navigating the yellow ADA wheelchair ramps at each street corner. By the time we'd gone two blocks, I was out of breath. Then I had an idea—get the wheelchair going faster as it went down the ramp at the first corner so that there was some momentum for going up the ramp across the street. On the first try, I trotted behind the wheelchair as I pushed it a little more quickly down the first ramp. I didn't see that there was a flaw, a two-inch lip at the front edge of the ramp across the street. Once the chair's wheels reached that lip, it was as if we'd hit a brick wall. Lee was launched forward into a standing position, but I was able to lunge over the back of the chair and grab his belt at the back of his jeans. At the same time, people nearby gasped loudly and reached for Lee, too. I pulled back on his belt with all of my might to keep him from being thrown to the ground. The sudden jerk on his belt made Lee plop down hard in the chair.

"Are you OK?" I yelled.

He smiled wide and said, "Sure!" as if he thought that slam into the seat was part of the ride. I immediately buckled the seat belt over Lee's lap, having learned a valuable lesson.

The wheelchair turned out to be a lifesaver as we waited in line to enter the stadium at the disabled guests' entrance. Lee enjoyed people-watching the time away. As I'd hoped, we were late enough to be spared the loud warm-up music on the field but early enough to watch the team run out.

After our seat neighbors and I got Lee situated in his seat, I took the wheelchair to a chain-link fence not far from the entrance. A month earlier, I'd received the permission needed to lock the chair there with a metal chain and padlock I'd brought along. Apparently, my request was the first of its kind for that stadium.

Lee was thrilled that he was at the first home game of the season, which warmed my heart, but the experience was extremely tiring for him. By halftime, he asked to go home. After one more game, Lee told me that he didn't want to go to games anymore, and we gave up our season tickets.

I'M DOING FINE

I think that accompanying Lee to doctors' appointments was one of the most trying tasks I did as a caregiver. I almost always went home choking back tears.

At a follow-up appointment with his cardiologist, the doctor asked Lee if he slept OK.

"I sleep really well," Lee said.

I knew that by this point he slept for three or four hours, then fitfully after that. So, I told the doctor what I knew about Lee's nighttime sleep habits. Then the doctor asked Lee how often he had to get up to go to the bathroom.

"Never," he said.

"Do you have trouble urinating?" the doctor asked.

"No," he said.

I bit my lip this time. Lee had instinctively started sitting and leaning his upper body forward over his knees to help him be able to urinate.

Then the doctor asked Lee if he exercised. I had to fight to keep from choking at that question. Lee said nothing and looked at me, his signal that he wanted me to answer for him. I explained that I had dropped Lee off at the front door of the doctor's office today, then parked the car while he waited for me in the lobby. Then we took the elevator together, and by the time we reached the office door, Lee was huffing and puffing. The doctor said that we must not be able to go to any football games, then. (Lee's cardiologist was a big fan, too, and we had often crossed paths at games in years past.) Lee replied that he did go to the games, and the doctor looked impressed. As they chatted about the quarterback, I could tell that Lee felt proud that he had gone to the first game and that he knew a fact or two about the team's performance, too.

I said nothing about what it took to get Lee there, to a game. I was bumping up against the need to protect my husband's pride versus the need to convey the truth to a medical professional.

Then the doctor asked about Lee's eyesight. Lee said that he had good eyesight.

Waiting for a pause in the conversation, I interjected with a question: "Lee has severe cataracts and was told he will need surgery soon. Is the surgery advisable, given his cardiac history?"

"What are you talking about?" Lee said angrily. "My eyes are fine."

He read some words displayed on a poster at the far end of the room, and the doctor seemed convinced. Lee's performance was convincing to me, too. I don't know how he was able to read that sign, given that the ophthalmologist had said that he was legally blind as a result of the cataracts.

I kept my mouth shut for the rest of the doctor's visit and tried to do the same at other medical appointments.

SPELLS OF FATIGUE

As 2014 wore down, Lee's daytime fatigue became so bad that he started needing to sit on the edge of the bed for fifteen minutes after a shower, until he gathered enough energy to get dressed. Once he was dressed, he had to rest in his recliner for a couple of hours to recover from the showering and dressing. More and more often, Lee used my help to pull him up from his recliner to a standing position. He needed a walker but vowed to "hold out" on using one, saying he feared that once he started using the walker, "it will be all over."

By the end of the year, Lee lay in his recliner, resting with his eyes closed, for at least half of the afternoon. Occasionally, he'd opt to go to bed midafternoon, sitting up just long enough to eat lunch. Then, on December 14, 2014, Lee stayed in bed for the entire day. When he needed to make it to the bathroom, he asked for my help to get him up to a standing position, and after pulling him up by his belt, I held on to the belt to steady him behind the walker. He didn't fight using it on these very bad days. The neurologist and family-practice physician both said that there was nothing that could be done.

Once our husbands suffered from severe fatigue, there was an interesting phenomenon that my caregiver friends and I noted. When our spouses were around certain people whom they wanted to impress (usually certain family members), they "turned on" to somehow look as if they were in much better shape than what we saw day-to-day. It was as if Lee could pump himself up the way I used to do when I had small children and was ill with the flu. I'd just put my head down and dig deep, getting through the day somehow. Now, I was amazed at how Lee could "dig deep" when one of his kids picked him up for lunch. Once he was back home and we were alone, he'd collapse into the recliner or bed and sleep for hours.

Lee woke up on Christmas Eve 2014, excited about the

dinner party planned at one of his kids' homes. He was show-
ered and dressed by early afternoon; then I settled him down
for a nap in his recliner. Even though he tried to rest, he became more and more fatigued as time passed and eventually
asked me to cancel on the party.

"I don't think I'm up to going," he said.

"How about if we wait a while to see if you might feel better after resting some more?" I asked, wondering if he could
dig deep for a couple of hours.

A little while later, after I saw Lee struggle to make it to
and from the bathroom, I dialed his daughter's number and
handed the phone to Lee. He got right to the point, too tired
to ease into the conversation. A few hours later, Lee's younger
son dropped by on the way to the party so he could pick up our
gifts for the family. As I saw him to the door, he quietly told
me that, after seeing his dad's condition, he would have made
the same decision. Lee's fatigue was literally visible on his face.

The fatigue was making it harder and harder to find ways
to bring my husband little moments of joy. After brainstorming one day, I thought I knew a surefire way. For years, he had
talked about splurging to get his beloved classic 1970 Ford
F150 pickup repainted, but he had never pulled the trigger.
When I made the suggestion, Lee was thrilled and ultimately
decided to repaint it the same original Yucatan gold color.
Every day, he talked excitedly about riding in that truck once
the paint job was finished, but, when that day finally came, he
was too tired. After it sat all shiny in front of the house for a
week, Lee was finally able to take a short ride to show off the
truck to his twin grandsons. He smiled so wide and was so
proud! That was the first and last time Lee had enough energy
to ride in his beloved truck. Yet every time he walked in or out
of the living room, he stood at the large front window for a
couple of minutes, grinning proudly as he admired the truck
parked in front of the house. Lee's world had shrunk so small,

it was thrilling to him just to be able to look out the window at the truck sitting there.

Knowing what that truck meant to Lee, seeing how hard it was for him to move in and out of the house, and catching glimpses of him looking out the window at the truck several times each day, not one neighbor complained about the pickup being parked on the street in front of our house for years, accumulating leaves and dirt underneath. I continued to look for ways to bring my husband slivers of joy through the fog of his fatigue.

CHAPTER 5

2015

The sixth year after the diagnosis brought challenges that were nearly too much for me to bear as a caregiver. Late at night, I would break down into tears as I sat alone in the living room, begging God for help. Lee's family-practice physician began broaching the subject of palliative care. There was nothing more that could be done to help Lee's body now. I was beginning to have serious doubts that I could physically care for Lee to the end.

Friends advised me to turn to an outside caregiver agency for help in our home. My support group's leader, Jerri, went further, cautioning me to find a memory-care facility for Lee as soon as possible.

A CRISIS OF CONFIDENCE

On the morning of January 14, 2015, Lee was sitting in his recliner when he told me in a worried voice that he needed to urinate but couldn't and that the bladder pressure was killing him at that moment. My mind immediately turned to my uncle, who had also suffered from dementia and had lived in rural Georgia. Two years earlier, he had been unable to urinate but hadn't told anyone for three days. My cousin explained that by the time they got him to the hospital in Atlanta, the bladder issue had led to a cascade of body failures that ended with a fatal cardiac event. With this uncle in mind, I pushed Lee hard to try again. When he went to stand up, his legs buckled. For some unknown reason, he was unable to support his own weight on his legs!

I couldn't get Lee out to the car on my own, so I called the county paramedics to take him to the emergency room. Lee was terrified that something was terribly wrong, yet the anxiety made him fight going with the paramedics. It was decided that I should ride in the front passenger seat of the ambulance and talk with Lee as he rode to the hospital, which helped his anxiety a bit. A bladder scan ordered by the emergency-room physician looked normal, and Lee was able to move a little urine while there, so he was referred to a urologist and discharged. I was so focused on the bladder issue that I didn't think about asking the doctor how to deal with Lee's inability to stand on his own. A nurse wheeled Lee out of the emergency room; then she and I were able to get him into Lee's older daughter's SUV by lifting him by his belt and legs while he pulled himself up by a handle above the dash.

The more experienced ladies in my support group had warned about our husbands eventually needing Depends, a walker, and possibly even a wheelchair. I had decided to be as prepared as possible, purchasing them one by one during the last couple of years. Once at home, Lee's daughter helped me to get Lee out of the car and into the waiting wheelchair. At the front-porch stairs, we somehow supported and helped him up each of the three stairs, through the front door, and back into the wheelchair.

It was clear that Lee couldn't stand at all on his own, and

I couldn't lift him or support his weight by myself. And I had no plan. This situation was a caregiver's nightmare. When he announced a few minutes after getting home that he had to go to the bathroom, I panicked. Using sheer willpower, Lee did a sitting push-up against the arms of the wheelchair to raise his rear end up from the seat while I grabbed his belt tightly and somehow thrust him toward the toilet. He landed badly but was able to get himself situated. Somehow, we were able to get his pants pulled down.

Once ready to get up from the toilet, Lee fought with all of his might to get his legs underneath him, and by working together, we were able to slip his pants up and get him into the wheelchair, where he landed kind of sideways. Lee was going to get hurt if we kept doing this. There was no way we could manage to move him multiple times a day. Lee sat in the wheelchair for the rest of the afternoon, until we moved him one more time into bed. There was no choice but to put Lee in adult diapers at this point.

I started calling caregiver agencies first thing the next morning, and each agency in turn told me that they did not help care for people who couldn't at least stand up, support their own weight, and shuffle their feet. Immobile people presented too great of a risk to agency caregivers, they said, and it took more than one or two people to move the dead weight of a completely immobile person. Lee would need to go to a skilled-nursing facility, one that had a Hoyer lift, the agencies advised.

Luckily, the situation was a temporary decline. We made it the three days until Lee could stand on his own again, but the experience left me terrified. *What if this happens again? What other potential Alzheimer's situations are coming that I'm not prepared to handle?* My caregiver confidence was shaken.

The appointment with the urologist was a week later, and the symptoms were completely gone by then. The doctor compared a before-using-the-bathroom ultrasound to an after-bathroom ultrasound and found that while Lee couldn't completely void his bladder, it emptied well enough. The urologist warned that the problem might return in the future, since it was most likely caused by the Alzheimer's. He passed a follow-up recommendation to the primary-care physician, who prescribed physical therapy at home three times a week for five weeks to try to improve Lee's strength. Lee's primary-care doctor made the referral to a very good home-health agency for the physical therapy in our home.

A registered nurse from the home-health agency came to the house on January 23 to do a pre-therapy evaluation, and then the agency's physical therapist began visiting a few days later. This physical therapist was competent, funny, and compassionate, a real bright spot in our day. Eric had Lee increasing his flexibility in no time. And he even showed me how to handle the weak-leg situation if it ever happened again: by using a super-slick varnished wood board called a transfer board. We practiced using the transfer board twice with Eric's guidance, and I saw I could easily tuck one end of the board under Lee's thigh while he sat on the bed and then side-scoot him along the board from the bed to the wheelchair. We tried it again from the wheelchair to the toilet. It was such a relief to finally have a solution for the leg problem, if ever needed. I ordered a transfer board from Amazon that same day.

At the time, Medicare's rules dictated that to qualify for home-health care, the patient had to be a "shut-in." After a couple of weeks of physical therapy at home, Lee refused to continue. Now that he could walk again, he wanted to go out for rides and to restaurants and couldn't seem to understand the need for physical therapy. Lee just couldn't handle staying at home every day in order to qualify for home health, so the home physical-therapy sessions had to stop.

Although the therapist's instructions, advice, and

encouragement had given me a badly needed renewal of confidence, Eric warned that there would be a time when I wouldn't be able to manage caring for Lee on my own. I was a sixty-four-year-old woman with spinal and heart issues. After that conversation, I never stopped worrying that there would be other Alzheimer's situations in the future that I hadn't planned for, situations that could blindside us again.

NOTHING IS EASY

Lee had outpatient cataract surgery in May 2015. I had debated long and hard about whether he should have it, knowing that physicians discourage elective surgery for dementia patients. Lee already had a lot going on medically, too. Still, the ophthalmologist lobbied hard for the surgery, telling me that it didn't require general anesthesia or an overnight stay, was done in a surgery center instead of a hospital, would only take a half day from start to finish, and, most importantly, was badly needed. "It's a very easy surgery," he said. Lee's blurry vision was driving him crazy on a daily basis now, so Lee and I set the date.

The surgery prep was simple. The nurses encouraged me to sit next to Lee and hold his hand as he lay on a bed in the pre-op area. The nurses were helpful, joking with Lee every time they passed by. Lee seemed very relaxed. The most difficult part, he said, was lying flat on his back while waiting his turn.

The procedure only took an hour, and the post-op stay only required a half hour of sitting in a recliner, easy for him to tolerate. At first, Lee had a sense of humor about the patch over his eye, but by the time we got home, he had forgotten about the surgery and just wanted to rip that thing off his face.

With the help of some distractions, he did keep it on for the time required.

By dinnertime, Lee was adamant that he'd never had surgery as I tried to help him with the prescription eye drops. He threw things while yelling at me to leave him alone and stomped off. I had to nag for a long while before he'd allow me to put the drops in his eye. But the most difficult post-op struggle was when he wanted to rub his eye. The healing must have caused some itching, and we fought about that all day long, every day of the recovery. Each time he started to raise his hand up to his eye, I reminded him that he'd had surgery and asked him to leave his eye alone so it could heal. If he ignored me, I pulled down on his elbow to get his hand away. "I did not have any damned surgery!" he'd yell.

At night, I was supposed to fix a plastic patch over his healing eye with surgical tape to protect it during sleep, but of course Lee ripped the patch off within minutes. Once his right eye was healed, we went through the same process again a month later for his left eye. I prayed for the entire month that he wasn't messing up his vision with the noncompliance.

"It's a miracle!" he exclaimed after both eyes had healed, completely forgetting about the surgeries. "My eyes have changed, and I can see everything so clearly!"

For days he commented on the beauty of the sky, the flowers, and the people walking on sidewalks as we drove by. I felt that the surgery was definitely worth the experience.

The last post-op appointment was more difficult than the actual surgery. Lee was angry about having to wait quite a while in the reception area and then for another twenty minutes in the exam room. Everyone in the office could hear him loudly grouse—about how long he had been waiting . . . about how this office had no respect for patients . . . about how the doctor was just so pompous . . . and so on. The situation was mortifying for me. I prayed that it was obvious to people that Lee had dementia so that they might understand his loud venting, but at least one employee was clearly upset. I wished I had prewritten business cards in my purse to hand out: "Please excuse my husband. He has dementia and is not in control of his emotions, thoughts, or faculties. Thank you." A couple of friends had said that passing out these kinds of apology cards was really helpful. Instead, Lee and I received stares.

The technician finally came in to conduct a post-op eye test and quickly went through the first set of choices.

"Is lens A"—click—"or lens B"—click—"better?" he asked while flipping between two lenses.

After seeing Lee's pained face as he struggled with choosing, I asked if the pace of the comparison could be slowed down and explained why I asked. The technician gave me a dirty look but did. At the end of the exam, it was determined that Lee had twenty-twenty vision but would need glasses for reading for a while. From the optician's display on the other side of the building, Lee immediately chose new eyeglass frames, an easy choice since it was the only pair that he liked. I jumped to order the glasses and get him out of that office as quickly as possible. I'm sure the staff were all relieved!

A couple of weeks later, Lee picked up the mail from the mailbox, opened the bill from the ophthalmologist, then loudly objected.

"What is this charge? I've never had eye surgery! Where are these eyeglasses we're being charged for?" . . . and so on.

I knew that he had to go back into that office one more time to get the frames fitted to his face and held my breath when we did. By then, Lee had forgotten about the bill and that he'd had surgery and was thrilled with his "miracle vision" as he was fitted with the reading glasses. I discreetly slipped a check for the new glasses to the optometrist and another one to the front office for the prior visit. The entire experience was unbelievably exhausting, but it seemed worth it now that Lee could see well again.

HONESTY

During the weeks that followed the eye surgery, I began to notice that Lee's overall condition appeared to go downhill. He must have noticed, too, and was running out of patience. One afternoon, I caught him starting to open a pill case and suspected he was making an attempt to feel better. All of our medications were quickly relocated to a more secure location.

At the next neurologist's visit, the dosage of one of the Alzheimer's medications was increased, and it seemed to make Lee even more tired. After a few days of the daylong fatigue, Lee volunteered, "My brain feels weird. This part behind my forehead, it just feels confused. I can't shake it. I just don't know what to do with myself." He asked me point-blank, "Donna, what's going on?"

I was shocked by his physical awareness at that moment, by his ability to communicate in detail about his body, and by his apparent openness to hearing the truth. None of these had been present for a long time, and I felt at that moment that I had to be honest, but I also knew that Lee could easily be overwhelmed. And it made no sense to give him information that might traumatize or upset him if he was going to quickly forget what I said anyway. So, I started out small.

"Alzheimer's makes people tired, and it sometimes makes it hard to get out of bed," I carefully offered.

"I already know that," he fired off with a frown.

"You don't have to get up in the morning, you know," I continued. "You can stay in bed for as long as you want, even all day! I can bring you breakfast, lunch, and dinner in bed, like you're my rich Lord Leland." I curtsied deeply at the front of the bed, and he laughed.

I had been struck by the impulse to somehow get the point across that at some time in the future, Lee might not be able to get out of bed, but that I would never leave him even if that situation came to pass. My attempt seemed to go well; my husband quit asking questions. I think he'd been after that very reassurance. All the same, after that conversation, he pulled himself out of bed by 9:00 a.m. to greet the day and to look for me.

NEGOTIATING AN EMERGENCY

In the spring of 2015, I woke up at 2:00 a.m. with my heart flopping crazily in my chest. I had lived with significant arrythmias since I was twenty-nine years old and did a pretty good job of self-diagnosing whether it was just benign premature ventricular contractions (PVCs), which were common for me, or something else more serious. I'd received a cardiac ablation in 2006 that had nearly eliminated supraventricular tachycardia (SVT) episodes and could recognize that arrhythmia. And the pacemaker seemed to help quite a bit to keep my rhythm more regular. But once every couple of years, I'd end up in the ER because of an unusual, scary arrythmia. Tonight, I thought I needed to be checked and called 911.

"Could you please ask the paramedics to turn off their sirens in my neighborhood?" I asked the dispatcher, explaining that my husband with Alzheimer's was asleep.

While answering her follow-up questions, I wrote out a note telling Lee that I would be back by lunchtime (but not mentioning where I was), then put it on the dining-room table with a cereal box, bowl, spoon, and sugar bowl. (I sent up a quick prayer that I'd be back by noon.) I also left a note on the coffee maker saying that it was broken so Lee wouldn't try to use it. Grabbing my purse, I quietly closed and locked the front door behind me.

Just then, the ambulance pulled up to the house, and a paramedic got out.

"Did you call for us?" he asked, looking perplexed.

"Yes, I did," I said, stepping up into the wagon. "My husband has Alzheimer's, and I'm trying not to wake him."

"We've never had a drive-by pickup before!" he teased as he connected the ECG wires to my chest.

Once in the ER, the doctor examined me and said that the arrythmia she saw right then wasn't dangerous but that I would need to be under observation for twenty-four hours. I knew that the observation period was part of the protocol the ER always had to follow for heart issues. It protected the hospital against liability in case something bad, like a heart attack, was on the horizon.

"I'm the sole caregiver for a husband with Alzheimer's," I explained. "Would you allow me to consent to treatment with one change: to drop the observation period if the usual second round of blood work, the X-ray, and the ECG all come back normal? I really need to get back home no later than 11:00 a.m., if I'm OK."

A nurse taking notes looked up at me with wide, surprised eyes and then locked eyes with the other nurse in the room. I almost laughed. I bet no one had tried this negotiation before. To the nurses' (and my) astonishment, the doctor smiled and agreed.

"We'll try to get the tests done as soon as possible," she told me. I had tears well up in my eyes as she left the room, thankful to have that ER doctor who understood what it meant to be a dementia caregiver.

The nurses teased me, saying that they wanted me to

negotiate their next car purchases! The crazy arrhythmia had stopped as soon as I'd arrived in the ER. After the second round of blood-test results came back as normal and my ECG and chest X-ray both looked fine, I was discharged. I called a cab and made it home by 7:00 a.m. Lee was still asleep, and I was overwhelmingly relieved.

CAREGIVER INITIATION

My friends had been getting more up front with their advice to hire a caregiver for a few hours in our home so that I could get my hair cut, attend doctors' appointments, shop, and maybe even see my grandkids without worrying about Lee's safety. I really wanted to spend time with my daughter during the up-coming Mother's Day. That desire pushed me to research rating websites, and I found an agency that seemed perfect.

The agency liaison suggested that I make a short first care-giver appointment to introduce the idea to Lee, to see how well a specific caregiver would fit with our situation. In fact, the liaison suggested that we try several caregivers until we found one who clicked with Lee, and I thought that was a great idea. I made a first caregiver appointment to get my hair cut and a second evening appointment a week later so I could go to Jerri's caregiver support-group meeting. When the first profes-sional caregiver appeared, Lee threw such a fit, yelling, stomp-ing around the room, and throwing the cable-TV remote and a book, that she had to leave before I could even get out the door. I was shocked at his behavior; this was nothing at all like the Lee I'd known. During the next couple of trials, I was able to get away from the house, but the caregivers had to call me back home soon after. The agency's rules required that their employee caregivers leave immediately if a client became ag-gressive, and Lee's shouting, threatening, and throwing things across the room were over the line for them. The caregivers never reported these outbursts to their agency, which would have caused it to drop Lee as a client. I kept thinking, *I'm just trying to run simple errands, for gosh sakes.* Lee's reactions seemed so over the top.

On Mother's Day, Ruth arrived. She was a little older than I was, a former Air Force nurse and the widow of a man who had succumbed to Alzheimer's. She'd been stationed in Turkey and Spain and tried to break the ice with Lee by asking about his years living in those countries. At first, he reacted as usual.

"If you leave," he told me, "I will divorce you. I don't need any damn babysitter!"

"I know it's a sacrifice for you," I said. "But Ruth isn't a sitter, she's a nurse."

"I'll run away!"

"Please, Lee. Can you please let Ruth stay as a Mother's Day gift for me? You've told me for eighteen years how much you love me. Now you have a chance to show me."

He listened intently, but a moment later, he'd forgotten what I'd said.

"I don't need a babysitter," he repeated.

We went round and round like a broken record. Finally, Ruth stepped in. She was one of the few caregivers who'd actually read Lee's agency profile. Best of all, she was an expert caregiver. By the time I'd eased myself out the door, Lee was telling her about his assignment in Seville, Spain. This was the first time I'd been able to leave the house without guilt or worry.

My daughter and I had a wonderful six hours together on that Mother's Day; it felt like a breath of fresh air. Lee wasn't mad at me when I got home. He told me that he really liked Ruth! She was perfect, an absolute gem. Of course, after an hour or so, Lee forgot about Ruth but still remembered that I had left him.

"Promise me you will never hire a caregiver again," he pleaded.

That was when I made the biggest caregiving mistake of all time—I didn't book Ruth immediately for a set day and time each week. I thought it was better if I just hired Ruth as needed, for Lee's sake. By the end of the following week, the word was out about this new caregiver, and she was booked solid. I was only able to have her back three times after that. That misguided attempt at reducing the caregiver impact on Lee haunted me. In the long run, it would have been much kinder for his sake if I'd just booked Ruth ahead for every week. Trials during the weeks after with new caregivers were disasters.

A few months later, we met Sandy. She was in her late sixties and a retired dessert chef who had worked at a four-star hotel in Los Angeles. Sandy was patient, intuitive, and hardworking, trying to win Lee over by baking him cookies and pastries. Once I was gone from the house, Lee usually calmed down enough to simply put on a passive protest, lying on his bed, staring up at the ceiling, and refusing to eat. Yet the outbursts when Sandy first arrived and as I left the house were an entirely different matter. Sandy ended up witnessing some extreme scenes, without flinching. She told me that she wanted to stay because she felt sorry for me, and, unbelievably, she never told the agency about Lee's behavior. We had an unspoken arrangement: Sandy would immediately call me back home if Lee scared her or if he didn't calm down soon after I left. If Lee did calm down once I was gone, I was able to get out of the house for a couple of hours. I started relying on Sandy's advice on the best ways to extract myself from the house, and she helped me through several scary situations. I must admit that the entire process was disturbing and exhausting for both Sandy and me—and for Lee. I would be shaking by the time I left the house and have nightmares for nights afterward.

For Sandy's, Lee's, and my sake, I didn't book her unless I absolutely had to. Sadly, after three or so months, Sandy had to tend to her own husband's worsening health issues, and we lost her. I was back to square one, trying to find another caregiver I could trust.

FAMILY

In years past, I'd taken my grandkids on all of the typical fun grandparent outings: to the museum, the movies, the park, and so on. Those outings died away as Lee's disease progressed. In 2014, I'd tried babysitting preschooler Eli for a couple hours once a week while my daughter volunteered in the older kids' classrooms, but even that minor distraction stressed Lee out. Eli was a quiet child who entertained himself at Grandma's house. Arranging toys for the three-year-old in the den and then running back and forth between grandson and husband, trying to give each of them attention, was impossible. Lee couldn't tolerate my spending more than five minutes in the den with Eli before he would urgently yell out my name.

In June 2015, my son and granddaughter came to visit from California. At first, Lee sulked at the disruption to his routine, but he eventually did adjust, not wanted to embarrass himself in front of our houseguests. I was uplifted by having this fun time with my family! That same summer, my younger daughter and son-in-law visited from Colorado, too, staying at my older daughter's nearby house so that their visit would be easier on Lee. My daughter was seven months pregnant with her first child and very excited to show off her "baby bump." I went to a baby shower put on by my daughter's local friends and to dinner with them afterward while Lee's younger son stayed with his dad at our house. I have to say that week was exhilarating and heartwarming.

After these visits with my family, I was now acutely aware of what I was missing and determined to find a way to get time away to be with my family. Yet Lee fought even more stubbornly at having agency caregivers in our house. I was always the one who gave up the struggle, and in hindsight, that was a huge mistake. I can never get those years back with my children and grandchildren.

On August 4, 2015, one of my cousins in Georgia called to let me know that another cousin in Florida, one who was ten years younger than I was, had died unexpectedly from a brain hemorrhage. The news was a shock and devastating. This phone call began a gut-wrenching decision-making process that went on for the next twenty-four hours. *Is there any possible way I can make it to the funeral?* Both of my parents were gone, and this deceased cousin and his parents had been my closest extended family members. I called my aunt Anne, and, true to character, she seemed more worried about me than she was about her own loss. She had friends and family with Alzheimer's and knew well what Lee and I were up against. In the end, Aunt Anne made the decision for me.

"Lee needs you at home right now; you need to stay with him," she advised, as we both cried through to the end of the call. I missed my family so much, my heart ached.

HYGIENE

Most new moms stop experiencing squeamishness after a dozen dirty diapers and a few of their babies' spit-up episodes. Twenty-five years later, I learned that dementia caregiving would rid me of any remaining queasiness. All of the hygiene rituals healthy adults do in private will, at some point, become a caregiving activity, too.

At the urging of the more seasoned caregivers in our

support group, I had purchased incontinence underwear well in advance of the need for them, just in case. Lee had experienced his first bladder accident on the way home from his cardiology appointment in July, but to protect his pride, I waited to see if the problem continued before suggesting he wear the underwear. It didn't.

During the summer, Lee also complained about his scalp being itchy. Ostensibly to ask him a question (but really just to observe), I popped my head into the bathroom as he took a shower. It was astonishing to see him rubbing his hand over his hair and body but with no shampoo or soap or washcloth anywhere to be seen. Lee took me up on my impromptu offer to help him with the itchy-scalp problem and loved the feel of a comb lightly passing over his scalp through a puffy lather of shampoo. The weekly "spa treatment" was a hit, and the itchy-scalp problem soon disappeared.

A few weeks later, Lee accidentally turned the hot water *up* instead of *off* as he tried to get out of the shower. He needed help showering from then on. I bought a shower chair with adjustable legs. Even though it barely fit in our shower, that chair turned out to be one of the best caregiving purchases I ever made. While sitting on the chair, Lee enjoyed my soapy scrub of his body and then couldn't wait to use a newly installed shower wand sprayer—it was really like being in a spa now, he said. Because he was preoccupied while sitting on the chair, I was able to turn the shower on and off without him grabbing the faucet handles.

Lee's shower routine was now a two-person endeavor, but it didn't take long, and he really enjoyed it.

GOOD DAYS

For one entire week in August, we experienced days that were unusually good. Lee was able to go to church, go out to lunch, and go out to breakfast with his buddies during that week. I wondered if he'd have occasional good days from now on or if this was an isolated upswing that would end at some point and not be repeated. I encouraged Lee to come up with ideas for outings, fearing that this might be his last chance at doing some of his favorite activities. I have to admit that the upswing was exhilarating for me, too.

On the eighth good day in a row, we left home to run a thirty-minute errand, but by the time we got to the destination, Lee could barely walk. I helped him back into the car and reclined the passenger seat so he could lie back and rest. He wanted it left that way for the entire ride home and was clearly very disappointed at the sudden change.

Late in the morning on another good day, Lee asked to go to one of our favorite bakeries and appeared to be up to it. After we pulled into a disabled parking space, I helped him from the car and, as always, took hold of the back of his belt to steady him as he walked up a curb. All of a sudden, Lee recoiled from the curb edge as we approached it, then gingerly extended the toe of his right shoe to feel around. I talked him through stepping up onto the curb the way I might have done for someone who was sight-impaired. It appeared that Lee had suddenly lost his depth perception and couldn't differentiate visually among the street, curb, and sidewalk.

On another promising day, Lee insisted on going to his favorite breakfast place, but by the time we had traveled the ten minutes to the location and parked, he said he needed to rest in the car. Once he felt able, Lee got out of the car, but every time he tried to let go of the car's door handle and walk toward the restaurant, his legs buckled. Without saying a word, I pulled the wheelchair out of the back of the SUV. (Luckily, I'd left it there after the last use.) Then I navigated it to just behind him and waited. Eventually, he gave up and sat down.

After three or so weeks of these energy-level swings, we got into a routine of watching out for the occasional good days and taking advantage of them as fully as possible. There was no way to predict when they would occur or how long a good day's stamina would last. We also couldn't predict the degree of difficulty of each bad day that came along. Lee quickly forgot the specifics about each good day in August before the sun would set on it, but that taste of a more normal life seemed to leave an impression on him. I prayed that we would see more. My life as a caregiver had to be completely "go with the flow" now.

QUANDARY

Late on the morning of September 21, I saw Lee grab his upper left arm as he walked to the car after breakfast out. At first, I assumed it was related to the physical-therapy session he'd had earlier for a "frozen" shoulder. Then, a nagging unease came over me. *Is it shoulder pain?* I wondered. *Or is it a heart problem radiating pain into his arm?* The pain went away once he was resting in his recliner at home, so I dismissed my suspicion. An hour later, after Lee got up to go to the bathroom, his upper left arm started hurting again as he walked.

"Can I call a doctor to ask advice on how to help your arm pain?" I asked.

Lee rolled his eyes but relented. The doctor asked me to give Lee a nitro pill while he stayed on the phone. When the pain immediately stopped, he advised, "You need to hang up and call 911."

Lee didn't argue. After an ER exam, he was moved to an inpatient room to wait for a cath lab procedure. The room had large windows that revealed a broad expanse of sky and the rooftops of nearby hospital buildings. The doctors weren't going to do the procedure that night, so Lee was given half a turkey sandwich and then, toward nighttime, a light sedative. He was calm.

I was beyond exhausted, so once Lee drifted off, I left to go home, stopping at the nurses' station to tell them that I had tried to teach Lee where the call button was on the bed remote, but he couldn't remember. I'd also written a note about using the call button on the whiteboard in his room but doubted he could read the board from the bed or understand the note. A nurse assured me that they would check in on Lee often throughout the night. After calling a cab from the lobby, I arrived home at 12:30 a.m.

At 8:00 a.m. the next morning, I found Lee in his room laughing with the floor's nurses. One nurse explained that they had forgotten to turn on the bed alarm, but Lee had been able to get himself to the bathroom without any problems. It was a relief to see Lee doing so well!

A few visitors showed up throughout the morning and afternoon with get-well cards and balloons. Lee basked in the glory of their attention. In the late afternoon, he dozed while *Gunsmoke, Bonanza,* and *The Rifleman* played at low volume on the TV. Our clergyman came by to pray with Lee, and he appreciated that visit, too. There were other effective distractions every so often, like when Life Flight medic helicopters occasionally landed on a nearby rooftop in view through the large window across from his bed.

Lee was taken to the cath lab at 5:30 p.m. and returned to his room at 7:00 p.m. When the cardiologist spoke with me out in the hall, he was more straightforward than ever before. There was nothing more that he could do for Lee's heart, he said. This was the same news I had been given after Lee's widow-maker heart attack. But I was confused. Yesterday morning, when I had called Lee's doctor, he had told me to call

911. I didn't stop to think about the fact that this advice conflicted with the cardiologist's prior advice. And getting help for a loved one was a habit so ingrained in me that I didn't know how to do anything different.

Lee had survived a first heart attack and quadruple bypass twenty-five years earlier, plus multiple catheter procedures since then.

"While last year's three stents looked fine today, the quadruple bypass done in the 1990s is pretty well blocked now and can't be fixed," Lee's cardiologist explained.

He then went on to explain that other blood vessels that had been stented over the years weren't looking much better. Even more very small blood vessels were blocked but could never be stented.

At least the cardiologist had taken Lee into the cath lab and double-checked that there was nothing more that could be done.

Lee was ordered to lie flat on his back for four hours, until 11:00 p.m., so that the puncture of the major femoral artery in his groin could heal. But by 9:00 p.m., he was starting to get impatient, unable to see the TV when lying flat. Trying to head off an episode of agitation, I asked the nurses for his routine bedtime antianxiety pill and for something soft to eat. I knew that if he didn't get that dose of medication very soon, I was not going to be able to keep Lee calm. They finally crushed the pill into applesauce, raised his bed a touch, and fed it to him. Lee dozed until 10:30 p.m., at which point he started insisting on getting up to use the bathroom. I was able to stall him until 11:00 p.m., the time he was allowed to sit up, get out of bed, and go to the bathroom.

On the way back to bed, the situation changed on a dime. Lee started looking very anxious and insisting that he had to go home. I tried to explain where we were and why and that the doctor wanted him to stay overnight. In a defiant fit, Lee ripped off his heart-monitor leads, saying that he had the right to check out of this "hotel" if he wanted to.

"I'm a grown man," he shouted. "No one can make me stay!"

I pushed the button to call for help, and two nurses quickly entered the room, but we couldn't stop Lee from pulling out his IV line. Then he tore off his hospital gown and looked around frantically for his street clothes. Completely naked, Lee moved toward the window.

"Why did you put me in this nursing home?" he asked.

I tried soothing statements. Nothing worked.

"Where's the exit?" he shouted, still buck naked and feeling around the windows for a handle. "I'm going home!"

The nurses tried to talk him down, too, but quickly realized that it wasn't going to work. When two male nurses entered the room, it was crowded. I slipped out of the way, taking a seat as far from the tumult as possible, leaning forward to hide my face in my hands to try to avoid seeing whatever happened next. I think the four nurses got him flat on his back on the bed while an injection was given to calm him. They sounded concerned and determined, yet not surprised. After the drug took effect, nurses re-dressed Lee, reinserted his IV, and pulled a blanket up to his chin.

Lee had "hospital-induced delirium," I was later told, which is not uncommon when dementia patients are hospitalized, they added. The scene was so unbelievable, I could no longer tell myself that Lee's case of Alzheimer's wasn't that advanced. This episode had stripped away all of my denial.

At midnight, when I was fairly confident that Lee was asleep, I told the nurses I had to leave. My arrythmia was really acting up, and for some unknown reason, my heart was beating very hard in my chest. It felt as if I would end up in the hospital myself if I didn't get some rest. I gave Lee's nurse my phone number and told her I'd be back in the morning.

"I just can't come back until then," I said. "I'm too exhausted."

"Can you give us some other family members' numbers, too, just in case?" the nurse asked, and I did.

I got home by 2:00 a.m. but couldn't sleep, what with the recall of the delirium episode crowding my mind. And with my heart beating so very hard in my chest, it was impossible to relax. An hour after eventually falling asleep, I was awakened by a call from the hospital. The medication had worn off and Lee was out of control again. They asked if I could come back. I told the nurse that I physically couldn't make it, apologized, and hung up, then immediately fell back to sleep.

I made it back to the hospital sometime between 8:00 and 9:00 a.m. and was walking down the hallway to Lee's room when I overheard him making demands in a loud voice and then a family member giving it right back to him, calling Lee "demented." I had a hunch that this family member had probably been called by the hospital immediately after I was called at 3:00 am. It was obvious that Lee had pushed this family member well beyond his limits.

As soon as I stepped into the room and noticed the family member's clenched jaw, I said, "Go home; I'll stay for the rest of the day." He flew out of the room.

Lee was demanding to go home. I explained that if he left "against medical advice," we would have to pay the entire hospital bill, which after a cath-lab procedure would be in the tens of thousands of dollars.

"The doctor has to sign you out," I repeated, "in order for the insurance company to pay anything."

That financial threat did the trick, and he lay back on the bed, albeit completely dressed in street clothes, with his shod feet hanging off the side as if he were poised to get up and walk out any minute. I ordered his breakfast and was eventually able to help him scoot up in bed and eat. Afterward, he was much calmer.

Not long after breakfast, Lee's cardiologist appeared. We talked out in the hall and discussed that a lack of food, the strange surroundings, plus fear and fatigue had been a bad combination last night, but that Lee looked much better today. The doctor reiterated that there really wasn't anything more that could be done for Lee's heart.

"Lee needs to be at home," the doctor said. "Can you manage him at home by yourself?"

"Yes, as long as I have instructions if I need to do anything new or special, and a few days' supply of any new drugs, if you or another doctor has prescribed any, so I don't have to leave him alone to go to the pharmacy."

The cardiologist nodded. To my great relief, Lee was discharged by noon that same day. At home, he collapsed into his recliner, ate a sandwich, and slept for hours.

The following day, I noticed a large, very dark bruise where the catheter had been threaded through an artery in Lee's groin. A couple of hours later, he noticed it too, freaked out, and didn't believe my explanation that he had gone through a medical procedure or even that he'd been in the hospital. Once I showed him some hospital paperwork, Lee relaxed and didn't bring up the bruise again. One day later, we were back at the Griddle for brunch.

At a follow-up appointment in November, the cardiologist told Lee that he didn't need to worry about going into the hospital ever again. He grinned, taking the doctor's statement to mean that his heart was healthy now. The doctor's expression when he looked in my direction changed from a big smile to convey a different message to me: I should not bring Lee into the hospital ever again for heart issues. I understood that nothing more could be done for Lee's heart and that it's wrong to take up space in the hospital when a case is hopeless. Others need the doctor's time. And some doctors had hinted that we needed to move to palliative care, working at keeping Lee comfortable but not taking measures to address any new medical issues. I was beginning to sense an unspoken suggestion that it was kinder for those with late Alzheimer's disease to die sooner from another medical condition than later from Alzheimer's disease. But no one had explained to me what I was supposed to do when Lee had pain in his arm or his heart or his hip or his gut, when he looked to me for help. Was I supposed to just ignore his complaints? I had no idea how to respond to medical situations now and was losing sleep as I worried about doctors' expectations of me if another medical crisis hit.

As a girl, I had attended K–8 parochial schools staffed by Sisters of Mercy nuns, an order that focused on nursing and teaching. My teachers were the most patient and loving people I'd ever known. I'd revered these teachers, and those instructing the upper grades often lectured to us about Mother Teresa and that it was our moral obligation to unselfishly care for others, too. Students heard that each person is here for a reason that is predetermined by God and that every person is valuable in God's eyes, regardless of his or her mental or physical condition. These lectures could be summed up in one statement I'd heard years later, a rendering of words penned by Martin Luther: God doesn't love us because of our worth. We are of worth because God loves us. And so, I grew up with the belief that loved ones deserved compassionate care regardless of their condition.

I had no idea what to do the next time Lee had chest pain. I just knew that I wasn't going to hurry Lee's death along and couldn't sit by to watch him experience pain and a fear of dying without doing something about it. Yet I understood where the doctors were coming from as they asked me not to bring a terminal case into the hospital or to look to them for healing help. I was in a deep quandary.

THE GAZE

There's a unique blank stare, an unmistakable facial expression that is prevalent among people with advanced dementia. Once I caught on to this look, it was like I'd discovered a key that allowed me to notice the Alzheimer's disease present in people all around me. (It was eerie when I'd meet someone in line at the grocery store, notice that gaze in the husband with her, and then have her whisper at some point that he had Alzheimer's disease.) I noticed that blank look in Lee for the first time at the end of 2015. Occasionally, he would sit in his recliner unaware of where he was. At times, he could barely walk. On one of those days when he had the empty gaze, I debated canceling my doctor's appointment at the last minute. It was obvious that Lee wasn't up to having a strange caregiver in the house in his disoriented state, and he definitely wasn't up to going along to my appointment or staying home alone. It took me a minute before I came up with the idea to call Lee's best friend, Bill, for help. I'd never called on him to sit with Lee before.

Lee was thrilled to have Bill over for a visit. I was, too, since Bill was a trustworthy, capable sitter, having cared compassionately for his late wife for many years as she suffered with cancer. When I returned from my doctor's appointment, Bill was near tears. I think it was too much for him, too heartbreaking for this sweet Southern gentleman to see his best friend in this state. I pledged never to call on Bill again.

Lee started talking often about seeing designs on his solid beige bedroom walls. Somehow, he knew that I didn't have the same vision.

"It must be caused by old age," he said.

I responded, "How creative. Can you describe the designs? Maybe we could redecorate your room to incorporate them?"

He laughed. Though they weren't scaring him, I knew Lee's visions were not a good sign. I started keeping more lights turned on to prevent shadows.

On December 15, Lee had the gaze and was completely disoriented. I had assumed he would never forget a place where he had lived for thirty years, but there he was, lost in the dining room. I was so grateful that this level of disorientation wasn't with him often.

BARRIERS

During the week before Christmas 2015, Lee's spirits were on an upswing even though he couldn't walk much due to back and hip pain. He began agreeing to let me push him around in the wheelchair, and we were able to get around fairly well. However, the three stairs from our front door to the sidewalk below were becoming a barrier to going outside the house. I called every business and handyman I could find online and contacted my caregiver friends for referrals. No builder contractor I reached would take on the project of building a ramp at the front of our house, saying the liability was too high. I wished that I had researched getting a ramp installed years earlier, before it was needed.

Eventually, I found metal ramps for sale online, ramps that were probably intended for loading equipment onto trailers. They would have to do. After setting up the longer ramp from the front door to the sidewalk below, it became obvious that the slope was too steep. It took all I had in me to push Lee's two hundred pounds up the ramp, and it was treacherous trying to control the wheelchair going down the ramp, too. In the end, using the metal ramp was such a challenge and so scary that we only used it a handful of times. I had a handyman build a sturdy handrail on the right side of the front porch's three stairs. On the bad days, Lee was able to lean on the railing and work his way down the steps without a problem. He was determined to get out of the house.

THE LAST CHRISTMAS

As Christmas approached, I badly wanted to take Lee to the mall to soak up Christmas cheer, a holiday activity we had always enjoyed a great deal. On his first good day in mid-December, when it seemed he might be open to riding through the mall in the wheelchair, I loaded my husband into the car, and we set off by early afternoon.

Lee and I watched children sitting on Santa's lap at Santa's Village, excitedly listing off their wishes. We took in the larger anchor stores' window displays while listening to the beaming high-school choirs nearby. Lee suggested we choose gifts for each other, and we made our way into Macy's. In the middle of the jewelry department, with the smiling saleslady watching on, he pulled me down to his wheelchair level so he could hug me and tell me he loved me. For those few moments, it felt like we had stepped back in time to when our focus was on the love we had for each other and not on the Alzheimer's. I had tears in my eyes as we moved on down the store's aisle. That afternoon, surrounded by the sights and sounds of the season, was magical. Lee forgot about our trip to the mall within a few hours, but I never will.

The Sunday before Christmas, Lee was able to go to the children's special Christmas service at church by agreeing to use the wheelchair. Several of the kids in our family had parts in the service—the younger ones were singing Christmas carols, while the older ones performed speaking parts that retold the Bible's Christmas story. Two also played musical instruments. We took lots of pictures, and everyone got hugs all around. People in the church were good about treating Lee no differently from anyone else. He was obviously pleased to be a full participant in the festivities.

After the service, some friends and family helped to lift Lee up the stairs to stand next to the altar's Christmas tree. Then two of us took our places at his sides, discreetly holding Lee erect by his armpits while the rest of my local family members arranged themselves in a group around us for our annual holiday picture. When I look at that picture, my heart overflows. Later that afternoon, my daughter and her family came over for Sunday dinner. We all sat around the table, chatting happily about the kids' school projects and sports and about Christmas. The kids were beyond excited with Santa anticipation.

On Christmas Eve day, I helped Lee to shower after lunch and settled him into his recliner for a nap, so he'd be rested for the party at his older daughter's house. By 5:00 p.m., when it was time to get ready to leave, Lee was beginning to show signs of late-afternoon fatigue and expressed doubts that he was up to going. I thought he looked much stronger than last year, though, and I gambled that he could get through two hours of an early-evening party this year. In hindsight, I have to admit that I was pushing him to go because I suspected that this would be Lee's last opportunity to attend a party with all of his children, grandchildren, and great-grandchildren gathered together. Lee wouldn't remember that night's party for long, but his family definitely would. After I told him, "We don't have to stay long. We can use the wheelchair," he agreed to go.

For fifteen years, I'd done all of the gift buying for both of our families, and this year I made a unique gift suggestion one week before the party. Would Lee like to give his four kids keepsake gifts? He loved the idea. His mother (and later his sister) had held on to some of his childhood artifacts and then shipped them to Lee once he retired and settled in one place. There were also keepsake items from his adult life stored with the childhood items in boxes in the basement. I brought up the boxes and unpacked Air Force medals, elementary-school report cards, a crocheted tablecloth that his mother had made, and so on. He chose his eight favorites, and I carefully wrapped the gifts.

After the family finished with the Christmas Eve dinner, I set the eight wrapped gifts and a baggie with slips of paper numbered one through eight on the table in front of Lee, asking him to distribute the slips to his kids. He held the baggie out to each of his adult children, who pulled out two slips of paper each. The person who drew "1" on a slip chose first and unwrapped a gift. Lee naturally spilled forth with a story about that keepsake, and his story captivated us all. The same happened in turn for each of the remaining seven keepsakes. Lee was elated that everyone was enthralled with his stories and that the kids loved their gifts. They hugged their dad while genuinely admiring their new treasures, then gave me a heartfelt thanks.

By the end of the gift exchange, Lee was completely beat but happy that he'd gone to the party. His younger son helped to pull Lee's wheelchair down the icy sidewalk to our car and loaded his dad inside. On the ride home, as we passed by downtown buildings awash in colorful lights, Lee chatted happily as he relived the evening. That downtown scene was a magical way to end a special night.

We had been riding high on a wave of good days, and Lee was able to go to Christmas service at church the next morning. My daughter and her family had attended the Christmas Eve candlelight service the night before but joined us at the Christmas Day service anyway, so that we weren't there without family. Their extra effort made the service even more special.

Lee spent the remainder of the morning and early afternoon resting and was able to move around using his walker. We joined my family for an early Christmas dinner at my daughter's house; she filled the table with all sorts of delicacies. She is a much better cook than I am, and we all loved the dishes that she had prepared especially for us. After dinner, the kids showed Grandpa their loot from Santa and put on a little show.

The 2015 Christmas season was perfect. I was immensely grateful that Lee had experienced nothing but "good days" during that week, which made his participation in our traditional activities possible. As I had suspected, this was the last year that Lee was able to engage in the Christmas traditions he had always loved. I will savor these last Christmas memories for the rest of my life.

A NEW LOW

Lee's good days during December 2015 spurred me on to make a December 30 appointment for a haircut. On that day, the agency sent Mary, who told me once I got home that Lee had allowed her to sit in the den and peek in on him every so often. He was even willing to watch TV from his recliner in the living room while she was present. I was heartened by this news, that he was able to relax for a while even though she was there. Mary went on to explain that during the last half of the appointment, Lee instructed her to stay out of his sight. Even still, the situation wasn't awful.

Although it was a blessedly uneventful caregiver session that day, Lee refused to talk with me afterward. At one point, he insisted on calling his son.

From the next room, I could hear him say into the phone, "Tell Donna to never bring another caregiver into this house again."

This was the third or so conversation with his younger son about this topic over the last several weeks. As I left the room, I only overheard a little of what Lee was saying but guessed from what I did hear that his son was yet again patiently and painstakingly explaining to Lee why he needed a caregiver. Unlike during the other calls, Lee grew impatient and frustrated, shouting at his son and slamming the phone down. I had never heard Lee speak to his family that way. He refused to eat dinner and went to bed mad. I was shocked that Lee was still mad the next morning. Even though he wanted to go out to brunch, he continued to give me the cold shoulder.

During the afternoon, a friend of mine came by for a visit. We rarely had visitors, and I was really excited to have some social time. Amanda and I had worked together for many years, doing the same job but on different projects. Three months after I retired in 2013, my former manager had asked if I would consider working remotely. I needed the mental stimulation and could use the income, so I said yes and worked when Lee napped or went to bed early. Amanda now worked part time remotely, too, and I hadn't seen her in months. She was a breath of fresh air, an energetic and creative person who moonlighted as a part-time fashion and concert photographer. Even though she had been over to our house before, Lee reacted badly. He scowled at Amanda and asked me who she was, then walked by us every few minutes to glower at me. I finally realized that Lee didn't believe she was a friend; he assumed she was a caregiver. It was embarrassing for me and, I suspect, uncomfortable for Amanda. She didn't stay long.

After my friend left, I turned on a football game for Lee and got busy with housework, trying not to show how upset I was. For the first time since Lee's diagnosis, my situation felt hopeless. Leaving the house, regardless of how good the reason was or how little time I was gone, felt more and more punishing to the both of us. And I was realizing that having friends over for a visit was nearly impossible. Lee's disease was effectively cutting me off from the world.

The live TV coverage on New Year's Eve from Times Square, with its cheering and animated throngs, was a glaring juxtaposition to the quiet solitude of our living room as I watched alone. I remembered back to New Year's Eve 1999, when Lee and I reveled downtown at the huge street party hosted by our city to usher in the new century. We'd had so much fun, and it was exactly how I loved ringing in the New Year. Viewing the Manhattan crowd and remembering past New Year's Eves made my current situation feel even more dismal; I had to turn off the TV. That evening was the most depressing holiday I'd ever experienced in my nearly sixty-five years.

By the end of 2015, I desperately needed help. Lee was unable, even during his best days, to manage his own basic life activities now. And his "bad days" could be debilitating. My husband needed a responsible adult with him at all times. Because he fought outside help and reacted badly when my friends or family visited, I was completely isolated now.

CHAPTER 6

2016—The Move

I was stuck between a rock and a hard place. There were times when I had no choice but to leave the house—for my own doctors' appointments, haircuts, and food shopping (in the days before online was available). And I always hoped to join Jerri's monthly support-group meetings and an occasional Sunday service at church, but it was rare that I could. I tried a few times to take Lee along with me on errands, but he didn't have the stamina, even on good days. I knew that I needed to find a way to make the agency-caregiver situation work. It was the only way I could continue to care for Lee at home.

LEVELS OF DIFFICULTY

Later on New Year's Day, there was an urgency in Lee's voice and a distraught expression on his face when he announced that he needed to call his younger son. Unbelievably, Lee remembered getting short with his son and abruptly hanging up on him. I dialed the number and handed the phone to Lee, who immediately apologized to his son. After ending the call, Lee miraculously announced that he would be OK with having a caregiver at the house. Believing in his heartfelt announcement, I shared that I had a mammogram appointment in a couple of days. Lee reacted by quickly and loudly saying, "I don't need a damned caregiver!" as he stared straight into my eyes, his face set in a steely expression, and then adding, "I wish I was dead."

Lee refused to eat more than a couple of bites of dinner and then went to bed straightaway. Once the house was quiet, a flood of emotions hit me all at once—disappointment, frustration, guilt. Mostly, I was mad at myself for believing Lee's declaration that he was OK with having caregivers. I guessed I was never going to stop trusting what my husband told me, never going to remember that there was no real meaning in anything he said. I really needed to quit twisting myself up in a knot trying to get Lee to accept agency caregivers; there was no way that would ever happen.

A pity party set in hard; I fought back tears for the rest of the day, brokenhearted that our situation was not more like that of my close friend Betsy and her husband, Rich. Like me, Betsy wanted to be Rich's full-time caregiver to the end. Rich had been an optometrist and had to retire immediately upon receiving his Alzheimer's diagnosis. He kept busy at the gym, did yard work, and spent time with his family. After three or so years, he lost the ability to be active, to drive, and even to talk. Once Betsy felt he couldn't be left alone, Jim, a nonprofit's volunteer caregiver, spent every Tuesday afternoon with Rich, who never asked who Jim was when the volunteer appeared at the door. Rich didn't bat an eye when Betsy left him with Jim so she could run errands.

Betsy and Rich's sons also took turns two or three times a month sitting with Rich on evenings or weekends when Betsy wanted to attend Jerri's support-group meetings, a church event, or some other social engagement with friends. Her Bible study gathered one evening a week at her house, so she could continue joining in.

Betsy eventually also took Rich to an "adult daycare" at a memory-care facility for an afternoon once a week. He loved the chance to be social, never noticing the deficits of the others or that Betsy had left him alone in a strange place. Later, when Rich became weaker and could no longer go to adult daycare, Betsy hired an agency sitter to come to their house for three hours a week in addition to Jim's weekly visit. Rich never noticed when Betsy left him with these caregivers at the house.

When Rich fell and couldn't get up, Betsy called the neighbor across the street, who worked from home and who was happy to help. Several other retired neighbors also offered assistance. If these neighbors weren't available, her son quickly ran from work to help.

Once it got too difficult to take Rich out for doctors' appointments, Rich's medical care was managed by a home-health agency, with at-home visits at least once a month.

Betsy's daughter-in-law, a registered nurse, also stopped by every morning (after her night shift at the hospital and on her days off) to check in on Rich and to help Betsy with dressing him. Once it became necessary, she also helped Betsy to shower Rich. By that point, one or the other of the sons stopped by each evening to help Betsy change Rich into pajamas and get him into bed.

During the last ten months of Rich's life, a hospice-care agency's nurses, physical therapists, certified nursing assistants, social workers, and other professionals managed Rich's hospice care. As his condition degraded, one or the other from the team was at Betsy's house for two hours four days a week, and they encouraged Betsy to get out while they were there. Betsy and Rich's sons and daughter-in-law continued to provide support at the beginning and end of every day. Finally, during the last two weeks, family members took turns sitting with Rich around the clock so that he and Betsy would never be alone.

Because Rich was "go with the flow," never showing signs of anxiety or stress at being cared for by caregivers and medical professionals in their home, Betsy was able to keep up with her errands and outside relationships.

Although Jerri's support group had never played the "who has it the worst" one-upmanship game that some caregivers like to play, the group knew that Rich and Betsy's situation was as good as it got. Betsy knew it, too, and often said that she felt very blessed. I had two aunts with Alzheimer's who, from stories relayed to me, were also on the less difficult side of the dementia spectrum, going along with caregiver suggestions and seemingly oblivious to the unfamiliar people around them.

If I had played the comparison game, I am certain that Lee's case of dementia would have fallen onto the difficult end of the spectrum. Yet his was not the worst case I knew of. Years later, the husband of a relatively new member of our support group was expelled from five different memory-care facilities because of his extreme agitation and outbursts. Another man I knew of threw a chair through a large glass window at a facility in a fit of frontotemporal dementia agitation. Whenever I heard of a new diagnosis, I always hoped the person's case would end up on the less difficult side of the spectrum.

EPIPHANIES

Lee needed a routine fasting blood test first thing one cold morning in January 2016. He never minded blood tests, joking that he had become used to getting shots "by the dozen" when on active duty in the Air Force, especially right before a deployment overseas. Just in case he might become anxious at some point, I always kept the promise of a brunch afterward as an incentive to go. After the blood draw, the nurse put a stretchy gauze bandage around Lee's arm at the elbow, a common practice for patients on blood thinners.

Once we reached our usual table at the Griddle, Lee began to take off his jacket, then stopped and stood there like a statue in the middle of the restaurant.

"Why is there a bandage around my arm?" he asked loudly.

"You just had your blood drawn for a test, Lee," I said quietly.

"No, I didn't," he said, raising the volume of his voice. "Tell me what this thing is on my arm!"

When I noticed that most everyone at the tables around us had a kindly, sympathetic expression, I was less stressed as I tried to deal with the situation while standing there in the middle of the restaurant.

"I promise, we just went for your blood test. Please sit down, Lee." I reached over to take the bandage off, hoping that would calm him down.

"I did not have a blood test!" he shouted. "I don't believe you!"

I lowered my voice even further. "Why would I lie?"

Grudging acceptance and then fear crossed his face. Lee sat down and looked depressed for the rest of the day.

This was one of those moments when Alzheimer's disease smacked Lee in the face, when he had a cruel epiphany, when it was obvious even to himself that he was losing touch with reality, and panic overtook him. At these times, he was forced to face the fact that his memory was failing. I never knew when one of these epiphanies would happen, when I wouldn't be able to find a way to gloss over or mask the reality of his disease. Blessedly, these insights were fleeting.

THE CLOSING WINDOW

None of the agency caregivers who had been in our home ever reported the agitation and outbursts to their agency, although I'd had several caregivers leave in a rush when Lee started yelling and throwing things at me. One called my cell phone before I'd made it a mile away from the house and told me to come back home. She was waiting in her car, parked in front of the house, when I drove up.

"I felt like it was unsafe, like I had to leave the house," she told me.

Jerri kept harping that I had a window to get Lee placed in a memory-care facility and that it was quickly closing. She predicted that the situation with Lee's agitation was going to reach the point where I couldn't handle him anymore. The situation would not remain the same; it would get worse, Jerri advised. If I didn't move him into a facility soon, none would accept Lee, and I was going to be in a fix.

In January, as I walked toward the front door so I could greet a caregiver as she came up the front sidewalk, Lee went toe-to-toe with me in the entry hallway. He was obviously very angry over the caregiver's arrival. Suddenly, he widened his stance, braced his arms, and clenched his fists as if he were getting ready to punch me. His stature, especially his height, felt suddenly very threatening. It was terrifying standing there, even though I believed the likelihood of him actually hitting me was low. I instinctively screamed, which surprised Lee enough that he dropped his fists.

I couldn't find a way to effectively communicate this fearful entryway episode to anyone, not to family or friends. I'm not sure why I felt the need to share the experience, but I kept struggling to put what happened into words. That difficulty with communicating a frightful or traumatic event is probably why some new mothers struggle to explain what their childbirth experience was like, why combat veterans don't bother trying to share what they've been through with nonveterans, and why domestic-violence and sexual assault victims have such a hard time reporting what they've experienced to police officers. But once I described the situation to Jerri, she completely understood, and that helped me immensely. She had witnessed these kinds of dementia outbursts at the facility that she had managed years ago. She kept repeating her advice: it was time for me to move Lee into a memory-care facility.

A couple of weeks later, in February, Lee saw me curling my hair in the bathroom, sensed right away that I was getting ready to go out, and started yelling and trying to hit me with his cane. His agitation went on and on as the appointment time came and went. The caregiver never showed up. This situation had never happened before, where there was no natural conclusion to an outburst, either by my leaving the house if a caregiver was willing to stay or by our mutual cancellation of the appointment.

When I stated, "She's very late. I don't think the caregiver is coming," it had no effect on Lee. Trying to reason with a person who is incapable of reasoning doesn't work. After twenty minutes had passed, I ran into the bathroom and texted my manager to tell her I wouldn't be at her lunch meeting set to begin in five minutes.

Lee had worked himself up into such a tizzy that he stormed out of the house, walking north and then turning east down a street that led to a nearby cliff. That street was very narrow at first as it rounded a curve and was without a curb or sidewalk. As he traveled along the street's right edge, which neighbors used as a walking and biking path, I followed single file behind him. Every so often, he'd stop, turn around, yell at me to go home, and swing his cane in my general direction as a protest to my following behind. While I was somewhat worried about Lee stepping or stumbling in front of a passing car, which would typically come within just a few feet of walkers, I was terrified about the cliff one block away.

At one point, I stopped for a couple of minutes to see if that would cause him to stop, too, but Lee continued on, walking as fast as I'd seen him walk in a long time, fueled by an anger that hadn't diminished.

Jerri and an Alzheimer's Association instructor had separately recommended that caregivers take videos of outbursts as a tool for communicating with families and physicians. When I'd remembered that recommendation earlier, while still in the house, I'd taken a short video in the hallway. While on the side of the road now, I pulled my phone out again just as a car drove by. It was so close, I could have reached out and touched the fender, which scared the heck out of me. When I looked up to see if I recognized the driver, I saw that he was staring hard at Lee, who at that moment was swinging his cane at me. I was mortified. *How crazy this scene must look to that driver,* I thought, and wondered if the driver was a neighbor, one I might see in the future.

As I pushed the record button on my phone and worked through my embarrassment, I was struck by how similar the scene before me seemed to slapstick skits like *The Three Stooges* I used to watch as a kid. Only this time, it was an old man swinging an object at a gray-haired old lady instead of Moe swinging something at Larry. I couldn't help but laugh at the thought, which infuriated Lee. While trying to stifle myself, I continued to beg him to go home. Even though the bout of laughter was irritating to Lee, it was a blessing to me. That *Three Stooges* breather helped a lot to lower my stress level. This situation I found myself in *was* crazy.

Hoping that the experts were right, that the video I'd just recorded would convey the situation more effectively than I could in words, I immediately sent it to a family member while standing there on the side of the road. Because I didn't take the time to send a text with the video, the family member had no context for the situation. In the end, the video didn't help at all with building understanding. Instead, the recipient chastised me later for giggling "at Lee," without commenting at all about the outburst. It was hard not to feel completely abandoned and defeated.

About a half block before he reached the cliff, Lee got tired and turned back. The caregiver arrived an hour late, at the same time that Lee and I reached the front sidewalk. He immediately went into the house and to bed without saying a word, too exhausted to register the caregiver's presence. I gave the caregiver my phone number, immediately walked out of the house, and drove off in my car, desperate to get away.

OPTIONS

As I drove away from home, leaving Lee in bed and the tardy caregiver watching TV in the living room, Jerri's advice kept rolling around in my head. On the spur of the moment, I decided to make a facility visit. Jerri was right: I needed to move Lee now.

This would be my second visit to a memory-care facility. A few months earlier, after another severe agitation episode, I had driven to a facility just a mile or so south of our house. I took Lee with me for that first visit, hopeful that he would realize what was at stake. I tried impressing upon him that if he didn't decide to go along with the occasional caregiver in our home, he would have to move into a facility. Looking back, I can't believe that I'd thought Lee could reason through cause and effect. Even if reasoning was possible, he would have soon forgotten that realization anyway.

Lee had agreed to go along on that first tour but then

insisted on staying in the car once we parked in front of the facility. I'd seen the inside of the assisted-living side of this facility when attending four Alzheimer's Association informational meetings there. But I had no idea what the memory-care side looked like or what services were offered there. Lee said he would be OK waiting in the car for the ten or fifteen minutes I thought it would take.

When the receptionist at the first facility found out that my husband was a prospective resident, she handed me off to the marketing manager, who wouldn't show me around until she peppered me with questions about Lee's situation. I quickly explained that Lee was waiting in the car and that I was only there to get an idea about the memory-care facility's services. She pushed me again to bring Lee inside, and I was less patient this time in repeating that he didn't want a tour right now. It seemed the manager could tell I was losing patience, because she quickly began giving me an assessment of Lee's condition based on just the few answers I'd given, saying that it sounded like Lee needed to be housed in the memory-care unit. Then this manager divulged that if residents didn't go willingly into the memory-care unit, they were medicated.

I no longer cared about seeing this particular facility or hearing what this lady had to say. But when she offered to let me walk quickly through the facility, I decided to take her up on the offer. I did want to see what memory-care facilities in general were all about. As we walked from the assisted-living side through a set of locked doors into the memory-care side, the furnishings and decor immediately changed from homey to that of a hospital. We passed a group of the memory-care residents silently being led to an activity room, and they looked to me like walking zombies.

"Are those residents unable to talk?" I asked my guide.

"Most of them can't speak," she answered.

Of all my friends' husbands with dementia, only two were noncommunicative. I wondered if these residents were being heavily sedated.

Driving home, I thought about the fact that this facility was considered one of the best in the area. *Is this really the standard for memory-care facilities in our town?* That question gave me a chill and a panicked feeling.

Later that day, an administrator from the facility called to tell me that it was probably too soon in the disease process for Lee to go to a memory-care facility. I wondered, *How does she know where Lee is in the disease progression without even meeting him?* The caller asked if I wanted a more detailed tour of the assisted-living side of the facility. As she talked, I thought about the fact that the assisted-living side was unlocked and that there was a bus stop right outside the front door. Then she slipped in the real reason for the changed recommendation—the memory-care section had no available rooms. I later found out through the grapevine that this facility had a habit of offering rooms wherever it had availability, regardless of the patient's needs. "Inappropriate placements" violated my state's assisted-living licensing rules. Between the statement about drugging new residents to get them in the door and now the attempt to place Lee where he obviously wouldn't be best served, I knew that I would never set foot in that facility again.

Now, months later, in February 2016, I drove to a second facility, hoping it would be nothing like that first one I'd seen. The administrator of this second location had a good reputation and had cared for a very difficult case I'd known about, a case of frontotemporal dementia. (From anecdotal information, I believed this type of dementia to be the most difficult when it came to outbursts.) The administrator gave me a quick tour, and it told me everything I needed to know about this place. The facility consisted of two long parallel halls, each containing a wall of doors leading directly into residents' rooms. Bridging the two halls, at the end opposite the entrance, was a large room that was used as a patient gathering area and staff office. The entire facility was painted stark white, the floors were made of linoleum-type tiles, and the staff was dressed like hospital orderlies. No one smiled. The residents' rooms were small and starkly decorated, with only a bed and a small bureau in each. The common area had a small TV with wooden chairs set to face it, but the room seemed more like a nursing station than a recreational room. The residents sitting there were not interacting at all. This place gave me the creeps. I couldn't move the man I loved into it.

I was home within the hour. After the caregiver left, Lee came out of his bedroom and wanted to talk. I was shocked that he remembered his earlier behavior.

"I can't handle having a caregiver," he told me, in a tone that sounded weak and like an apology. "It's too demeaning."

At that moment, I got a strong sense that Lee had been terrified when I'd left him, when he was separated from me. My heart broke for my husband. No matter what option I considered, it was either torturous for him or impossible for me.

A couple of weeks later, the next time a caregiver pulled up to the house, Lee said that he wanted to kill himself. This was a new reaction to the agency caregivers. That caregiver said that she wasn't supposed to stay if a client was truly suicidal, but neither of us believed that Lee was serious. We suspected that he was trying to coerce me into staying, in much the same way a child threatens to hold his breath if his mother begins to leave him with a babysitter. The caregiver told me to keep my phone nearby once I left the house, and I promised my errand would be as quick as possible.

To my happy surprise, Lee ended up watching TV with that caregiver and was even cooperative. When I heard this report, I was beyond thrilled and thanked Lee for being kind to the woman. He smiled and said the situation wasn't the caregiver's fault. I couldn't believe what I was hearing. Maybe the situation could be turned around, and he wouldn't need to be moved into a facility after all? I was so excited; my hands were shaking. Then, a few minutes later, Lee repeated that he wanted to kill himself.

I left Lee alone at home, asleep in bed, in order to attend the next caregiver support meeting. I described what had happened over the last four weeks and asked the group for their ideas on ways to deal with the agitation. They all, to a person, advised me to get professional help at a facility as soon as possible. Everyone knew the agitation wasn't Lee's fault and felt sorry for him, but they also believed I couldn't go on. I began researching the latest Department of Health and Welfare facility-inspection reports for our state. Jerri pledged to do research on facilities, too.

Family members took Lee to lunch, urging him to accept having caregivers at the house. They warned Lee that I was planning to move him into a facility if he didn't accept having caregivers, hoping that Lee could realize what was at stake. At that lunch, they asked Lee to choose the facility where he'd like to live. That was an unexpected new approach at trying to get through to Lee.

After his son dropped him back at home, Lee was beside himself. He would only eat a few bites at each meal, couldn't sleep, sank deeply into his recliner, and stared off into space with no desire to watch his favorite Westerns on TV. Every few minutes, he'd say something to the effect that he just couldn't choose. After two days, my husband looked like a shell of himself.

During his more lucid moments, he'd talk about moving to his Iowa hometown, where he could buy a home and live alone, he said. I showed Lee the website of the Iowa memory-care facility where his sister lived now.

"If you went there, you'd have the company of your sister.

You'd see your niece and possibly some old high-school friends. But Iowa is far away. Your kids and I wouldn't be able to visit very often. Will you please consider staying somewhere closer to home?" I asked.

Lee said nothing.

Over the next week, Lee never forgot about his assignment. He acted as if all the facts he knew and his feelings about moving into a memory-care facility were thrown into a big pot and stirred up every few minutes. He would draw out a fact or feeling at random, discuss it, then drop it back in. A few minutes later, he'd pull out another fact or feeling, discuss it, then drop it back in. Then he might draw out a fact he'd already raised, repeat his previous discussion, and then drop it back in. This went on for days. Lee got more and more depressed, withdrawn, and weak from not sleeping or eating much. In the past, Jerri had told our group that families should secretly plan out a move in advance. Make it quick and without warning, she advised. Now I understood why she said this approach was kinder in the long run.

Lee spent a week ruminating and forgetting, ruminating and forgetting. Then he began a campaign in earnest to stay at home, promising he wouldn't get upset anymore when a caregiver arrived. He begged me to trust him and swore that he would keep his word. I had to give it another try. Even if Lee still couldn't tolerate an agency caregiver, the stall would hopefully help him to regain some equilibrium and strength. I just knew he was headed for an illness if he didn't get some sleep and eat. When I told Lee that I believed his promise and would get caregivers instead of asking him to move, he gave me a big hug, completely relaxed, and mostly slept for days.

I told the family that I was giving up on the move to a facility—but that if it turned out that a move was necessary in the future, I was going to handle the situation very differently. The move would be made quickly, and I wouldn't tell Lee ahead of time. Lee's younger son volunteered to help if I decided a move was necessary.

I was delighted that the next caregiver to arrive at the house was male and hoped that his gender would make a difference with Lee. He chatted with Kevin for over an hour during the first visit. But after Kevin walked out of the house, Lee still became angry over having a caregiver. I was relieved regardless. As long as there was no agitation while the caregiver was present, this situation could work out. So, I pushed on and arranged a standing weekly appointment with Kevin. We got through the next three dates, and I was thrilled that Lee was continuing to tolerate Kevin without showing any agitation. He wasn't happy with me and refused to talk with Kevin now, but we could live with that. On the fourth date, Kevin was scheduled for 6:30 p.m. but called at that time to let me know that he couldn't make it. After several more no-shows, some with no excuse, I realized that Kevin wasn't dependable. Soon, the agency fired him.

When Sandy, the fearless former four-star-hotel dessert chef, appeared at the next appointment, I was relieved. Her husband was doing better, and she was back to work. I immediately booked her available dates, kept my fingers crossed, and prayed that this arrangement would work out. However, I knew that if her husband got sick again or some other issue prevented her from working, I was out of options. That thought panicked me.

IN OVER MY HEAD

"Lee, today is Mother's Day. You used to make Mother's Day such a fun day for me when my kids were living out of town by doing really nice things for me so that I felt appreciated. You've always understood how important the holiday is to me.

I would really like to spend the day with my daughter. Would you like for me to do anything for you before I leave?"

I felt like I needed to give Lee a two-minute notice because I was leaving for the entire afternoon, longer than I'd ever left him with a caregiver before. He didn't seem upset. I set a sandwich and brownie on his TV tray. But when Sandy walked up the sidewalk, Lee yelled that I was not going to leave him. I could clearly see that he was panicked. As I opened the door and greeted Sandy, Lee grabbed my wrist in a flash and held on like a vise, twisting my arm while pulling me close to him. I was in excruciating pain. Sandy and I yelled at Lee and tried to get my arm free.

"You're hurting me!" I said with tears streaming down my face.

He finally realized what he was doing.

"I'm sorry for hurting you," Lee said, his expression looking tortured as he eased up just enough for me to yank my arm free.

In the past, I would have sent Sandy home and skipped my plans if something like this had happened, but I couldn't keep doing that. I was beginning to recognize that if I didn't spend time with my family once in a while, I was completely ignoring my own needs. I think Lee could tell that I wasn't going to give in this time. He grabbed a cane, then walked out the front door and down the street, taking the same route he'd traveled three months earlier, toward the cliff. I assumed he'd get tired before he reached the edge and turn back, as he had done before. In this case, Lee was full of adrenaline, moving quickly. Without hesitation, he soon reached the cliff and explained as he walked to the edge that he was going to take a shortcut, to run away. As soon as I heard the phrase "to run away," I realized that he was not rational at all and became terrified that I was not going to be able to keep Lee from tumbling down the hillside.

A narrow roadway had been carved into the steep cliffside from the highway below, curving up to our neighborhood on top of the hill. The cliff was made up of sand, rock, sagebrush, and wild grasses. There was no way anybody could get down that sheer side without sitting on his rear and falling or sliding until he reached the road below. As he stood on the edge but before he could tumble down, I grabbed Lee's belt at the back of his pants and pulled with all of my might away from the cliff. Lee began fighting my grip.

Just seconds later, my daughter walked up behind us and said calmly, "Hi, you all." She knew instinctively to underplay the situation, trying to keep Lee from reacting to her voice. He stopped fighting, backed away from the edge, and turned toward home. The real Lee, the man I had married, the man who was too much of a gentleman to act out in front of family, had reemerged. I was never so grateful to see my daughter as I was that day.

Sandy was still waiting at the house, and I hugged her.

"Thank you so much for telling my daughter which direction we'd gone and for waiting here. As soon as Lee heard her voice, he turned right back toward home."

Lee went straight to bed. Sandy thought that he would be calm now that he was so tired and advised me to go ahead with my Mother's Day plans.

"Keep your phone nearby, just in case," Sandy cautioned.

I knew Sandy was violating her agency's rules by not leaving the house immediately when Lee had grabbed my wrist. To be honest, I expected her to report his behavior this time, but she never did. Sandy and I agreed that Lee's agitation was caused by fear. Neither of us held his outbursts against him.

From Mother's Day through early summer, Sandy and I experienced more frightening events together, approaching them as partners in caregiving. She instinctively, deeply understood dementia and was able to look beyond the disease and truly grasp what Lee was going through. Yet while Sandy was a compassionate, effective caregiving partner, she believed that the day was quickly approaching when she could no longer work with Lee. She began to encourage me to find a memory-care facility right away. I was getting in over my head, she warned.

I had always trusted that Lee would never hurt me, because doing so would contradict the character of the man I'd married, a man who never, ever would have raised a hand against me. But after the delirium episode in the hospital, Lee's son had told me that his sisters had been advised not to be alone in a hospital room with their dad, a fact that had placed the first tiny little doubt in the back of my mind. And then there were Jerri's periodic reminders to keep our purses and keys in locations where we could grab them and make a quick exit from our homes, if needed. The further the disease progressed and the more out of control the agitation episodes seemed to become, the less trusting family members should be, she said. I knew deep down that the experts were right; I was in over my head.

THE DECISION

It had been five months since I'd backed off on the decision to move Lee, and the situation had not improved in the least. Then one midsummer morning, something clicked. Out of the blue, I decided I had to move Lee into a facility and soon. I don't know if my survival instinct just kicked in or if I plain wore out. I don't know if it was a recognition that I couldn't handle my husband's outbursts alone anymore or if I finally realized the impact of isolation on my life.

Jerri had repeatedly told me that it would be tricky moving Lee into a facility at this point. State licensing rules prevented any type of facility from accepting residents with serious agitation behaviors. It was imperative that I find a memory-care facility with expert staff, one that would know how to help keep Lee's agitation from becoming serious. I had to find a place that was capable of earning Lee's trust. It was also imperative that I feel at a gut level that the facility would protect my husband. On top of all of that, Lee was the most challenging type of resident: extremely intelligent, unbelievably stubborn, fiercely independent, and completely incompetent.

Jerri advised me to tour several facilities, to resist letting pretty interiors or fancy activities turn my head, and to trust my gut, making note of any red flags. She recommended that I look for a way to just sit in an out-of-the-way place without being noticed so that I could watch how the residents and staff interacted. Then Jerri gave me a list of four facilities in the area that she believed had competent, compassionate administrators. Two of these facilities had already been crossed off that list, but I still felt buoyed by her encouragement and advice.

I booked a caregiver for the midafternoon, steeling myself against the reaction it would elicit from Lee. The third facility on the list was just west of our house. I didn't call ahead, wanting to see how it appeared without advance notice. *How did I pass by this facility every time I drove to my daughter's house, a place located just three minutes from home, and never even notice it?* I wondered.

Unlike the hospital-type environment of the two memory-care facilities I'd previously toured, McMillan seemed truly welcoming right as I walked in the front door. Posters about upcoming activities hung over a console table in the entry. The living room to the left had a high vaulted ceiling that was underlined by a knickknack ledge. There was a huge stone fireplace tucked into the left corner of the living room, and in the right corner was an upright piano. In the middle of the wall, between the fireplace and piano, was a large TV that just happened to be playing a Western movie. Couches were scattered around the room.

"Is there any way I could have a tour of this facility? I'm looking on behalf of my husband," I asked a staff person who walked near the entry and glanced in my direction.

"You don't have an appointment? Our director is out. Gee, I will have to see if that's possible. Why don't you have a seat here in the living room?" she replied.

This is the best possible scenario. I settled back in a corner chair and just soaked in the body language of residents and staff members. There was an almost constant parade up and down an open hallway in view, where the residents and staff often stopped and talked with each other. They were within sight and most within earshot of me. I noticed right off that they seemed to interact comfortably. One staff member gave a big hug to a resident, who then smiled wide. Another staff member ran down the hall, speaking into a two-way radio. Residents asked questions or made requests of staff members, who responded immediately. I felt at ease in this place and, for some unknown reason, thought of my grandmother's house.

The assistant director appeared after four or five minutes.

"I'm sorry I've kept you waiting. I'm afraid the director isn't here right now, but I can give you a quick tour, if that's OK?"

"Thank you very much," I said while smiling wide, beginning to feel some hope.

It was impressive that she'd made the effort to help and was willing to squeeze an unscheduled tour into her day. We walked together through the living room and then into the adjoining combined kitchen and dining room. I began taking mental notes. *Look at how shiny and spotless the tiled dining-room floor is.* Bright-colored plastic tablecloths covered six long tables surrounded by eight chairs each. Landscape-style art hung on the walls. Small vases with two or three fresh flowers each served as centerpieces. *They make an effort to have a welcoming dining room for the residents,* I added to my mental notes.

A fifteen-foot-long half wall covered by a peninsula countertop defined the boundary between the dining room and the kitchen at the right. A resident was standing at that counter, joking with the cook, who was fixing him a snack. *The residents can snack whenever they want, and the cook sounds really nice.* The cook smiled and waved at me, and as I waved back, I noticed that there were pots boiling on the large industrial stove along the kitchen's back wall. A pantry door to the left of it was partially open and revealed stainless-steel shelving full of canned items. A moveable stainless-steel island in the middle of the kitchen held salad fixings on chopping boards. Sinks lined the left wall; two large industrial refrigerators lined the right. The kitchen looked organized and clean. *They make real food here for the residents and offer fresh produce, instead of serving reheated frozen meals.*

Three residents were seated at a dining-room table, happily chatting while a staff member brought them coffee and cookies. I also heard laughter coming from a room located off the other end of the dining room, and we walked over to peek inside. Residents sat at a long table in the "activities room," playing bingo. Most of them appeared to be very intent on winning. In the left corner of the large room, I saw dolls, brushes, and combs lining a dressing table, where a staff member was curling a female resident's gray hair. Two male residents were relaxing in recliners facing the right corner of the room, watching a show from the 1960s on a TV mounted on the wall. A popcorn machine sat nearby. Large windows and two open French doors looked out onto a patio. On the other side of the patio, I saw a grassy area with lawn chairs, shrubbery, trees, and two raised wooden garden beds. *This facility is so homey. The residents seem to be free to choose what they want to do, and they seem engaged and happy.*

ENDURING   137

I wasn't listening much to what the assistant director was saying.

"What type of room would you like to see?" she asked, cutting into my concentration.

"I don't know," I answered honestly.

So, she showed me all of the different configurations, which was surprising given that only one type of room was available on that day and that she was squeezing my tour into her schedule. There were two-bedroom, one-bedroom, deluxe studio, and regular studio units. People could double up in the two-bedroom units to save money, and that was required for those receiving Medicaid payments, the assistant director told me. There were only three double rooms in the facility as far as I could tell.

On this day, only a deluxe studio was available. It was spacious, with two large windows that looked out onto a gazebo on the front lawn and to the street beyond. The light gold-yellow of the walls was almost exactly the same color of paint as that on our home's living-room walls, the color I'd learned was best for those with Alzheimer's. The unit had a little kitchenette, with a dorm-type mini-fridge tucked under a six-foot-long countertop that included a sink. And there were cabinets above and below the counter. Two good-sized closets and Lee's armoire would provide plenty of storage for clothing. There was plenty of room for Lee's recliner and television to create a little sitting area. The bathroom was large, with lots of grab bars around, an emergency pull cord by the toilet, and a spacious walk-in shower with a handheld showerhead, just like at home. *I could live comfortably here,* I thought. This space was pretty much perfect.

The director of McMillan, Taylor Davis, joined us. She was a gracious, well-spoken woman in her late twenties or early thirties who had a really upbeat, positive attitude. As we chatted, I could tell she was very knowledgeable about dementia.

Later, I learned that she had several degrees in gerontology-related fields. Taylor seemed compassionate and gave me a strong sense that she really cared about her residents. As she spoke, I became convinced that this facility was the best possible place for Lee.

In Taylor's office, I wrote a check for the deposit and texted Lee's younger son at work to see if he or other family members wanted to tour the facility before I signed the contract. He immediately replied that he trusted my judgment. I completed the registration form, signed the contract, and gave the director the deposit check. Then we set the move-in date for a week later. As I left Taylor's office, I noticed a couple waiting on the other side of the office door, then heard them inquire about a place for their mom. *Lee and I have just experienced a miracle,* I thought.

THE MOVE

I knew that the decision I'd just made was life-altering for Lee and me. My hands wouldn't stop shaking at that thought. At the top of my mind was a determination to make this as smooth of a move for Lee as possible, and I knew it was going to take real planning to make that happen.

As soon as the caregiver left, Lee went to sleep in his recliner. I made my way to the den and closed the door, then quietly called Lee's best friend, Bill, who agreed to take Lee to breakfast at 8:50 a.m. sharp on moving day. Lee's younger son later volunteered to drop by the restaurant an hour after Bill and Lee got there. He would visit with the guys for a little while, then take Lee for a ride into the hills to see the aftermath of a recent wildfire, then drop it on his dad that he'd like to take a quick "tour" of the facility. This would give the movers and me around ninety minutes to get the furniture moved in and the room set up, and, most importantly, would provide a way to get Lee into the building.

Lee was still asleep after I hung up with Bill, so I went ahead and called a moving company, the one that Taylor had recommended. I could just picture Lee freaking out if a moving truck pulled up to the house while he was still at home. So, I asked if the truck could arrive at the house just after 9:00 a.m. the following Wednesday. The owner let me know that he had moved many other people into memory-care facilities in the past and promised that the crew and truck would wait around the corner if they arrived early.

I'm a list-maker, so I began one for the move. I needed to buy a new double-size bed frame, box spring, and mattress. We'd take Lee's armoire, bedroom television, clothing, trash can, and favorite artwork, four sets of plates and flatware, his favorite snacks for the fridge and cabinets, extra eyeglasses, linens and towels, and toiletries. (I didn't need to bring towels, it turned out.) Lee could no longer make it down the stairs to the daylight basement family room, so I secretly packed down there during his naps.

My support-group friends and out-of-state son bolstered me during frequent nighttime phone calls as I vacillated between guilt and determination. When I imagined Lee playing bingo or having coffee and cookies with the other residents, I felt convinced the move was for the best. When I reminded myself that Lee would have an RN watching over his physical health, which was becoming more and more complicated as time went on, I felt it was a needed change. Yet when I looked into my husband's eyes and kissed his face, I wanted to back out. I was on an emotional roller coaster. Jerri kept reiterating the fact that I really had no choice.

Before Lee would be accepted into the facility, Taylor and a registered nurse, Tanya, needed to interview him to assess how much care and assistance he would need. We made arrangements for a home visit three days after I signed the contract. On the day of Taylor and Tanya's visit, I told Lee that some friends from work were stopping by. Of course, he assumed they were caregivers and became stressed, which made me worry that he was going to have a meltdown at any second. But Taylor and Tanya effortlessly convinced Lee that they were indeed my coworkers and miraculously got Lee to relax within minutes of their arrival, expertly chatting with him and asking about his past. Throughout this seemingly casual conversation, they snuck in questions that tested his memory. Lee warmed up to them so quickly that he turned on his magnetic charm and beamed his adorable, dimpled smile for most of the visit. I stopped worrying about his agitation at the facility. The longer Taylor and Tanya interacted with Lee, the more convinced I became that he was going to be happy there and that they had the expertise to deal with his anxious behaviors.

Later, Taylor and Tanya emailed to say that they were excited to have Lee joining them and hoped his presence would encourage more men to move into the facility. (It did.) I felt God's hand intimately in what had happened over the last few days—in finding the facility, in discovering that the perfect room was available, and in Lee's response to Taylor and Tanya during the interview. That feeling of divine intervention helped to keep me strong.

After a couple of days, Taylor emailed to tell me that Lee's case was classified as Level 1 (of four possible levels). That was more good news. Level 1 meant that he required the least amount of care and would be charged the lowest monthly fee, $6,500. Unlike many other assisted-living/memory-care facilities in our area, McMillan charged a flat rate. They didn't charge extra fees for helping residents to shower, for dispensing medications, or for other services. Other wives had told me that these extra fees at some facilities could run into the thousands per month. The more services McMillan provided to a resident and the more time and help he needed, the higher the level of care, which increased the monthly rate. (The cost went up $1,000 per month for each increase in the level of care, to a maximum of $9,500 per month.)

Author's note: See the addendum at the end of this book, which offers a sample assessment that can be used to determine what assistance or level of care a person needs. It is a helpful tool for tracking a loved one's changing needs and for describing a loved one's situation and condition to physicians.

I emailed the names of Lee's doctors, a list of his medications, and a short medical history to Taylor and Tanya. They let me know that Lee could no longer receive his prescription drugs from our health insurance's mail-order pharmacy. All medications had to be from a special pharmacy in town that exclusively supplied drugs to facilities. This special pharmacy used a drug-storage system based on 8½-by-12-inch cards. Each drug's pills or capsules for one month were packaged on a separate card. So, for example, there would be an August card for Lee's thirty-one doses of Aricept. Each pill would be attached to the card in a separate and individually labeled little sealed plastic cup, called a "blister." So, on the fourth of the month, the staff member would look in the medication file for Lee's cards, find his Aricept card, and pop the dose from the blister marked "4th." This card system kept doses organized and secure and was required at all care facilities according to our state's licensing rules.

The facility also had a computer system that notified the medication technician when each medication dose was due. The med tech had to check off in the system anytime a medication was given to a resident. To me, this system seemed foolproof. We would now need to pay out-of-network costs for

Lee's prescriptions, making the $50 monthly expense jump to $400, but the safety seemed worth it.

The day before the move, I felt as prepared as I possibly could be. At the same time, I was sick to my stomach and full of dread. As soon as Lee went to bed for the night and fell asleep, I quickly moved some boxes into my car and dropped them off at the facility. I wanted an excuse to check that his new bed had been delivered and that his room was ready. Then I ran to a nearby department store to buy a new bedspread. My daughter had volunteered to shop for other bedding, towels, and supplies and had prewashed the new sheets.

On move-in day, Bill arrived to pick up his best friend right on time. My stomach was in knots as I kissed Lee goodbye, realizing that he was probably walking out of his home for the last time. I stood at the window and watched Lee walk down the driveway, then get into Bill's car. I couldn't make myself move from that spot even after they pulled away. That morning felt tragic; I fought back tears and nausea.

The movers appeared ten minutes later, and when I described our ninety-minute challenge, these young guys laughed and said, "Bring it on." They literally ran from the truck to the house and back again. Lee's things were loaded in no time; then I drove to the facility with their truck trailing close behind. The guys quickly brought the boxes and furniture into the room and arranged them into the floor plan that I had figured would make Lee most comfortable—one that allowed him to see the television from his bed and recliner. My daughter and I made up the bed; hung the curtain valance; placed Lee's ironed shirts, sweaters, and sweatshirts in one closet and jackets and blankets in the other; and then stocked the kitchen cabinets, refrigerator, and bathroom. The movers helped to hook up the TV and hang the artwork. We completely set the room up in eighty minutes! My daughter quickly left, and once alone, I couldn't stop my legs from trembling.

Taylor stopped by and complimented me on setting the room up in record time, then waited with me for Lee to appear. Just a couple of minutes later, he popped into view at the end of the hall.

"I've seen enough of this place," he was telling his son. "I want to go home."

Once Lee noticed me standing farther down the hallway, he stopped in his tracks and stared for a moment, then walked toward me. As he reached where I stood, Lee glanced toward the room's open door just a couple of feet from his right shoulder and saw his furniture inside. He knew without anyone saying a word and began to protest. Taylor immediately stepped between us, speaking gently. To my amazement, he gave her his full attention, quickly calmed down, and followed her. They were off to see something to do with the Air Force. As they walked slowly down the hall, Taylor motioned with her hand behind Lee's back, pointing toward the living room. I took it as her instruction to quietly leave. As soon as Lee was out of sight, his son and I quickly walked to the living room and out the exit door.

MCMILLAN

At the time I signed the contract and paid the deposit, I didn't realize just how lucky or blessed Lee and I were. Jerri had pointed me to a rare find among memory-care facilities. There were eight or so staff caregivers on duty at any one time caring for the forty residents at McMillan. They were young, in their twenties and early thirties. I don't think older women could have kept up with them. These caregivers dealt with a never-ending, constant swirl of tasks: helping this resident go to the bathroom, making sure that resident used her walker, helping most residents get dressed in daytime clothing first thing in the morning and in pajamas at night, assisting with toothbrushing, intervening in residents' conflicts, removing a resident from another's room, stopping a resident from rifling through drawers where he shouldn't, consoling someone who was confused or upset, getting a resident a snack, answering family members' questions in person and on the phone, cleaning up spills, re-dressing and possibly showering a resident after an incontinence accident, changing incontinence underwear on approximately half of the residents at least four times a day, making beds, helping in the activities room, collecting and cleaning dentures each night, serving and assisting residents with meals, cleaning up messes made by residents, and so on, and so on, and so on. The staff never sat down; they even ate their breakfast, lunch, and dinner while standing so that they could watch over their charges as they were eating.

These highly trained, intuitive women could sense a resident's stress or illness, often before families did, and alerted the nurses right away. They expertly redirected residents with agitation and were mostly successful. They came up with explanations for each resident with paranoia or anxiety that presented a kinder form of reality. And they fulfilled every resident's need or demand with patience, regardless of his or her grouchiness. It all seemed a bit unreal to me at first, as if they were putting on a show for guests, just too perfect. *Is McMillan a bit of a con game?* I wondered. After a few months, I gained trust; I was in the background and around the corner too often for any caregiver to be able to hide a mean streak or to put on an act. They were for real.

After some weeks it dawned on me that the staff members' high level of skill and dependable consistency was due to clear performance expectations, good hiring practices, and strong oversight from the lead nurse and the director. All of the staff were required to complete quite a bit of online and in-person training when they first began working at McMillan, and they continued taking online classes regularly. Some, especially the lead caregivers, had worked at McMillan for years. I think the most important reason for the staff's universal competency in caregiving was Taylor. By the end of a year, I'd seen a handful of new caregivers come and go, lasting for only two or three days once they revealed even a hint of snarkiness or laziness to another staff member or family member. It always got back to Taylor; we all knew she'd want to know. She loved her residents unconditionally and would not tolerate staff members who felt otherwise.

One senior staff member was always appointed lead caregiver and medication administrator for each shift. She watched over the caregivers, making sure they pulled their weight and lived up to the training. This person also had to be certificated in medication administration and stood like a sentry at her station in the living room, using a special computer program that prompted her to give each resident prescribed medications at specific times. Many of the residents were on blood-pressure meds, diabetes meds, heart meds, and so on. She had to preread any special instructions for each medication and each patient, while also watching for adverse reactions if new medications were given. The lead was also the coordinator of staff attention, using a walkie-talkie to get help for residents or visitors. If she had to leave her concierge-type computer desk, which was stationed next to the entrance of the living room, she called another caregiver in to temporarily take over her station for a minute or two, so she could find a resident who was due for a medication.

Added to the mix were two "activities" staff members who managed sing-along music sessions, bingo, exercise sessions, birthday and holiday parties, outings, barbecues, and other activities for the residents and who contracted with outside individuals and companies to put on weekly live music shows, monthly pedicures, and special movement sessions. They were on duty from 9:00 a.m. to 6:00 p.m. weekdays, moving the residents from one activity to the next. The cook on duty, the maintenance man, and the housekeeper were always available to help in different ways, too.

McMillan had one RN and one LPN. They buzzed around the facility, supposedly on duty from 8:00 a.m. to 5:00 p.m. on weekdays, but I could always find one in the building, working late for one reason or another. The RN, Becky, who was hired six months after Lee moved into McMillan, was so experienced, knowledgeable, and intuitive that she could tell immediately as she passed by a resident if something was off with him or her. She would stop in her tracks and take the resident to his or her room for a more in-depth examination if something didn't seem quite right.

Becky supervised all caregiving staff, leading rounds during shift crossovers, conducting in-person training at monthly meetings, and mentoring. She was the person who took doctors' orders and then updated the residents' medical records and the medication system to ensure they were followed. When an illness was suspected, she contacted families and physicians, then followed up on the prescribed treatments. The two nurses took turns being on call on nights and weekends, responding to staff questions, reports on changes in residents' conditions, and emergencies. They also responded to family texts and calls.

When I'd signed the contract for Lee's move into McMillan, I had no idea about all of the activities and the robust care there. I never stopped being thankful that Jerri referred me to that facility.

CHAPTER 7

2016—Adjusting

Lee had just moved out of the house when our twenty-year-old dishwasher gave out. The leak was bad and necessitated a disaster-cleanup company, requiring me to balance on floor joists as I grabbed items from the refrigerator. That weekslong project, with strangers traipsing in and out and large, loud fans running day and night, would have driven Lee to the end of his rope if he'd been living at home. I hoped the leak was a sign that Lee's move was meant to be and that he would be happy at McMillan.

THE TRANSITION

A two-week "transition period" began immediately after the move, a blackout of all communication between Lee and the outside world. Taylor told me that if Lee heard a family member's or friend's voice on the phone or saw us in person, it would restart a craving to leave and undo any strides he'd made in learning about McMillan and making new friends. She reiterated, all of the progress made adjusting to life at

McMillan—building trust with the staff and beginning new relationships with other residents—would be lost. Taylor was frank when she emailed me, "The new residents naturally think that when loved ones appear or call, they are coming to take them home."

I knew that Lee couldn't reason about the move. There was no quick way to help him accept living at McMillan. I understood the fact that he had to spend time there, letting the routine, his room, the fellow residents, the caregivers, and the place seep into whatever core memory he had left so that he could understand at a visceral level that this was where he lived now. Yet even though I agreed with the reasoning behind the blackout, I was going through a difficult adjustment, too. I missed my husband something awful and worried that he felt abandoned. To help me through this period, Tanya and Taylor sent me pictures every so often. One email included a video showing Lee smiling, eating cake, and watching a country singer perform live in the living room. I was surprised at how completely at ease he looked. That video helped quite a bit.

During the two-week transition, Taylor began brainstorming different "first visit" scenarios. Was it best for Bill to visit him first because Lee wouldn't insist that Bill move him back home? On the other hand, as Lee's peer, would Bill be put into a difficult situation, being pressured to take Lee elsewhere? Taylor decided to wait a few more days to make the decision.

Toward the end of the second week, Tanya let me know that Lee had made some friends and seemed to be acclimating very well, but that he hadn't accepted that he was living at McMillan yet. She and Taylor were now thinking that Lee needed a third week to adjust before the family visited.

"Lee is on a learning curve right now, getting to know his room, the staff, and the routine," she told me.

Taylor warned on another day that it was important for family to stay positive once they began talking with Lee, then ended her email by saying, "Thank you for all of your help in making this move so smooth for Lee. You are a great couple, and I'm sure that you both will work through this time of transition and remain a great couple." I cried when I read that last sentence. This transition was much harder than I had expected. I missed seeing my husband so much.

A couple of days later, when I made my daily phone call to ask how Lee was doing, the caregiver who answered the phone was obviously upset. *What could have gone wrong?* She spilled out that an earlier caller that day had insisted on breaking the blackout and had spoken with Lee. Because the landline phone's volume was set very high to help residents with hearing loss, she had overheard some of the conversation. The caller had told Lee that I should never have put him in McMillan and that "he was going to be there until the day he was carried out in a casket." The caregiver's voice cracked with emotion.

I did my best to try to calm this young staff member. After we hung up, I sat stunned, unable to understand why anyone would have made such a cruel statement to Lee. The only thing I could do was pray to God that he would quickly forget about the rogue phone call.

A few days later, Taylor let me know that I could finally see Lee. I was excited, hugging and kissing him when we first met! He wanted to complain instead, saying that he had no one to talk with.

"I shouldn't have to live here," he said.

I remembered the advice from Taylor to try to avoid getting into a downspin of complaints, so I quickly changed the subject. Lee soon forgot about his frustration once we were out of the facility—we needed to go to the ophthalmology office to get the cause of his new double vision diagnosed. It turned out to be caused by something simple: drooping eye muscles. That appointment was a blessing, because driving there and going together to a doctor's appointment made our time together during this first visit seem normal to Lee.

After the appointment, we went to a Sonic Drive-In and ate our lunch while sitting in the car, parked in their lot. That also seemed normal to Lee, to be eating burgers, fries, and chocolate milkshakes in the car. He looked very relaxed, which was a relief.

As we walked back into the facility, Lee saw his new friend, Mich, another Air Force veteran, watching a movie in the living room and was eager to join him. They soon were excitedly chatting away while sitting together on the couch. I learned that Mich had moved in just two days before Lee and then kissed my husband goodbye without any reaction at all from him. This first visit had gone so, so much smoother than I'd expected. I walked away feeling tremendous relief and exhilaration that Lee had a new friend to converse with.

The next day, Lee was fixated on his wallet, which he was now unable to find. I'd last seen his wallet on the day he moved in, when I'd put $200 in it.

"My pocket feels weird without my wallet," he complained.

Jerri had explained to the support group a year ago that men who were used to feeling wallets in their back pockets for decades almost felt as if a part of their bodies were missing when the wallets weren't there. So, I made a mental note to buy Lee a new wallet on the way home to replace the lost one. Thank goodness Taylor had warned me before the move to keep his debit card, DMV identification card, and health insurance card with me.

Later during the visit, Lee found an old wallet in his nightstand and slipped it into his back pocket. I could tell he felt better now, even though he didn't have his lost wallet back. This old wallet was empty, so I asked if he wanted some money for it. After I handed Lee forty dollars, he jokingly accused me of being cheap, then asked for his kids' phone numbers on a piece of paper so he could slip it into the wallet, too. Once he had the forty dollars and the paper tucked in the replacement wallet, Lee felt much better, more like normal.

An hour later, he proclaimed that his wallet had been found as he showed me the old one, which he had just pulled from his back pocket. The wallet crisis was over. Throughout the rest of that second visit, Lee tried to convince me that he would cooperate with having caregivers at home if he moved back.

"Lee, back in February, you swore to me with all of your heart that you would go along with having the agency's caregivers. But you just couldn't do it. I know you were sincere back then and that you are sincere now, but I also know that you need to be here."

I added, "Honestly, honey, with all of the medical problems and all of the medications that I was trying to keep track of and with your middle-of-the-night sleep problems, it's just too hard for me to take care of you right now."

Lee's face relaxed to a soft look. It felt so good to be having this heart-to-heart conversation about the move.

"Getting used to living here is stressful," he said, then paused, thinking. "But maybe the stress is because of the Alzheimer's?"

That admission shocked me. *Have the caregivers been explaining this to him, or is this a realization he's made on his own?*

"Yes, I do think the Alzheimer's is making everything much harder," I said. "And I feel for you. I really wish it didn't have to be this way, that you hadn't gotten the Alzheimer's."

Lee hugged me and let the topic drop. That conversation felt like we were clearing the air. I knew from experience, though, that any insights were probably short-lived, so I didn't count on this understanding holding.

On the third day, I asked Lee how he liked the food at McMillan.

"I hate it," he answered.

A little while later, I noticed a menu board just inside the entry to the dining room and learned that lunch had been tilapia and potatoes.

"How were the fish and potatoes today?" I asked a few minutes later, wondering if there'd be a different answer to a more specific question.

Lee quickly replied that he ate some fish and really liked the scalloped potatoes, and that he also had some pie, and it was really good, too. It was then that I realized my questions needed to be specific, or I would just get a general complaint.

On the way out, I saw Taylor, and she let me know that the staff had observed Lee mixing socially and doing activities with the group. She felt that Lee was adjusting well. It was such a relief to hear.

During the fourth day's visit, I took Lee to church and brunch, thinking it would be a good outing and bring him some feeling of normalcy. Lee only ate a couple of bites, telling me that he had been signed into McMillan for life and would only be leaving in a coffin.

On the fifth day, I showed up just before 5:00 p.m. to join Lee for dinner at McMillan, to see how he interacted with the other residents. Lee's appointed place was at the head of the table, the table that had the most functional residents assigned to it. He seemed genuinely excited, actually beaming, that I was having dinner with him. It seemed that all of the residents at his table were kind of excited, too, to have a guest at their table. They were quite conversational and animated as everyone took turns introducing themselves to me and sharing a little about themselves. *I would never have known that these folks have dementia if I'd met them in a restaurant,* I thought. Mich sat to Lee's left, and the two happily chatted about the places where they'd lived around the world.

By the time Lee had been at McMillan for one month, I could see the parameters of his good and bad days and felt I knew what to expect, at least for now. By this point, I had reached the conclusion that it was a very, very good decision to move Lee. The social interactions and staff support were having a positive effect on him, and his lows were nowhere near as low as when he was at home.

After two months, Lee settled into the routine at McMillan and seemed to feel comfortable with it. He even started to enjoy the monthly pedicures! Breakfast was at 8:00 a.m. sharp, lunch at noon, and dinner at 5:00 p.m., with no variation, ever. Sing-along sessions and bingo games were at the same time every day. This strict schedule provided an internal rhythm, a relief for those residents who had no sense of day and time.

The only area of contention that Lee seemed to have at McMillan had to do with showering. My independent husband fought hard against the staff's help, but they felt he needed it and didn't allow him to shower on his own. It was insulting to him, that these people didn't think a grown man could shower by himself. And he absolutely did not want the young female caregivers to see him naked. When I volunteered to help, the staff quickly took me up on it. The shower was very large, with plenty of room for his shower chair. His getting in and out was easy since there was just a two-inch lip separating the shower floor from the rest of the bathroom floor as well as grab bars on every wall. We soon got the routine down to fifteen minutes, and it felt natural after a couple of weeks.

An overall daily-visit routine also developed after a couple of weeks. Lee knew to expect me right after lunch and that I'd spend the afternoon with him. He settled down into a routine with Mich and the schedule at McMillan. There was a rhythm to life again.

RESPITE

After Lee had been at McMillan for two months, I decided to take a weekend trip to San Francisco, in September. The dear friends I'd made when I had lived in that city forty-seven years ago were planning a reunion, and I didn't want to miss it. The close proximity was a big selling point for the trip—one hour away by air. And my son worked in the city. He promised to get free whenever I had time to spare from the reunion. I couldn't wait to see him.

Lee's emotional situation was up and down during the week before the trip. After brunch on Sunday, he started hitting himself on the head as we drove back to the facility.

"I hate bingo!" he kept saying. "There's nothing to do there. I'm living with a bunch of crazies!"

"You don't have to play bingo, you know. Taylor and Krystal"—the activities director—"tell me that you and Mich hang out most of each day. And there are concerts and exercise classes, which is a lot more than you had to do at home. Plus, you have your own TV in your room, so you can watch your shows just as you did at home. It sounds to me as if you have plenty to do."

After we returned to McMillan and I had parked in the disabled parking space, Lee refused to get out of the car, insisting that I take him home. I put the keys in my purse, got out of the car, then stood quietly on the sidewalk near the front door. Eventually, Lee joined me, firmly stating that he was not going inside. After nearly a half hour of quietly standing on the sidewalk together, I walked to the front door and stood there. Lee got tired and eventually walked in. I left soon after.

A few hours later, a staff member helped Lee make a call to me. He wanted to apologize for the way he had acted. I couldn't believe that he remembered what had happened. His words of apology broke my heart.

I wrote an email to Taylor to ask if I should cancel my trip to San Francisco, and she replied right away.

"Your time away might be the best thing for you both," she wrote. "Don't worry, we'll give him extra attention and find things for him to do."

My flight back home on Sunday landed at 5:00 p.m., and I went straight from the airport to see how Lee was doing. After we hugged, he told me that he was dying to get out for a ride. A caregiver whispered to me that he hadn't eaten well while I was gone. As we pulled away from McMillan, on our way to Marie Callender's, Lee announced that he was never going back. I immediately realized that this outing was a mistake. Then I made the situation worse by deciding to go ahead and get him a sandwich anyway. *Lee is hungry, the staff member said. Maybe after eating, he'll feel more upbeat.*

The conversations of the other customers seated around us in the restaurant started driving Lee crazy. He began to get agitated and only ate half of his sandwich before insisting on leaving. Once outside, Lee refused to get in the car.

"I'm not going back to McMillan," he said.

After fifteen minutes of standing quietly on the sidewalk, I asked him to get in the car. He was getting tired and complied.

"You better not drive back to that place," Lee warned.

I quickly changed the subject to the flight's turbulence and to seeing my son and San Francisco friends . . . anything that might keep him distracted as I turned the car right out of the parking lot's driveway and onto the busy street.

Lee sat up very straight all of a sudden and said, "I know where you're headed," then opened the car door and tried to jump out as we were moving down the roadway!

He knew we were driving in the direction of McMillan as we traveled west on Fairview Avenue, a major thoroughfare with five lanes full of traffic. Time seemed to go into slow motion while my thoughts went warp speed.

"Lee, close that door! You're going to kill yourself!"

His shirt and jacket collars bunched together in my right hand as I quickly clutched at them behind his neck. Then I pulled him back and toward me. This threw Lee off-balance, like a turtle on its back, leaning him into me and away from the open door. I checked to be sure his seat belt was still fastened—it was—while remaining razor focused on keeping the car moving. I had a strong hunch that if we stopped, Lee would try to jump out again. Steering with my left hand while hanging on to him with my right, I drove without stopping until reaching the third corner. It had a red traffic light, but I didn't stop the car. With no cross traffic, I rolled the car through and made a one-handed right turn. After another four or five minutes of driving down that street and struggling to keep Lee off-balance, the car was closing in on McMillan's driveway. There was a center road divider up ahead that would block me from turning left into the facility driveway and parking lot. When I saw that there was no oncoming traffic, I steered the car onto the wrong side of the road and drove quickly into the parking lot. As soon as I shot the car into a parking space and stopped, I let go of Lee, and he jumped out and began walking as fast as he could toward the street, just as I'd feared.

I ran in the other direction, opened the facility door, and yelled loudly, "I need help!"

Caregiver Tiffany caught up with Lee in a flash and threaded her arm through his as she walked along with him, all the while sweet-talking.

"Hey, Lee, what do you think of the weather, darlin'? You were a weatherman before you retired, weren't you?"

He usually sweet-talked back with Tiffany, but not this time; he was angry, even with her. She said nothing more and just kept walking alongside him, arm in arm, to ensure he was balanced, I assumed. Eventually, Lee got too tired and gave in, following her back to McMillan.

I wondered if this agitation was Lee's reaction to my not visiting him for three days while I was in California. The next day, Taylor confirmed it, saying he'd been upset the whole time I was gone. Lee wasn't able to stand time apart from me, she said.

A LITTLE "OFF"

On October 19, three months after the move into McMillan, I got a call at 2:00 a.m. from Tanya, the facility's RN. She was calling from her home after having received a report from the night staff that Lee had fallen. The staff had examined him closely, she said, and he was fine, back in bed, going to sleep. I could tell that she didn't want me running over to see him, assuming that if he saw me, he'd never go back to sleep. Tanya promised to call if Lee's condition changed. I set my alarm for 6:00 a.m. and was up, dressed, and grabbing some cereal when my phone rang again.

"Lee looks . . . a little off," Tanya told me. "He should probably be seen by his doctor this morning."

It took me five minutes to make it to McMillan so I could see Lee's condition for myself. He was half-asleep or semiconscious, looking poured into an armchair in the living room. His eyes were so narrowly opened, they looked like slits in his face. I knew immediately in my gut that the situation was life-threatening. Tanya walked toward me, saying something, but I had tunnel vision, unable to hear anything she said. I never acknowledged her.

"How do you feel?" I urgently asked my husband.

He tried to reply, but his speech was so garbled and slurred, I couldn't understand him. Grabbing the cell phone from my purse, I called 911.

"I think my husband has a brain bleed or a stroke," I told

the emergency dispatcher. "He's on blood thinners and fell during the night."

"What is the address?" the dispatcher asked.

I gave her the name of the facility and the cross streets, unable to remember the street number. Then the dispatcher peppered me with questions about what had happened and when, his age, and his most significant health history. I took breaks from answering to reassure Lee and to put my arm around his shoulder.

"Hang on, honey," I said. "We're going to the doctor's office right away to get you help."

At one point, I looked up and noticed the night-shift caregivers standing nearby. They looked terrified.

While I was still on the phone answering the dispatcher's questions, firemen arrived from Station #10, located just a mile or so down the road. A firefighter EMT tried to get Lee to talk, but he still couldn't form sentences or stand up. In fact, he was barely able to sit up. I could tell that they were thinking this was something serious, too, as they examined Lee purposefully and took vitals with expediency. The paramedics arrived a couple of minutes later with their ambulance. As Lee was being loaded onto the stretcher, a paramedic and two firefighter EMTs stood facing me, staring hard.

"How long has he been like this?"

I explained, "I just got here, so I'm not sure. He fell at around 2:00 a.m. The nurse who called me at the time told me he was fine, uninjured, back in bed, and going to sleep. She called again fifteen minutes ago to say he looked 'a little off.'"

The EMTs and paramedic looked at each other and rolled their eyes. The nurse stood fifteen feet back from us and said nothing.

As I walked beside the gurney out to the parking lot, a caregiver ran out with a list of Lee's medications. With tears

in her eyes, she told me that she was so sorry. She was the one
who had found Lee on his bedroom floor.

"He'd crawled toward his bedroom door and yelled for
help after he fell," she explained breathlessly. "We got to him
right away."

This young caregiver warned me that there was a streak of
blood on his carpet from where he had scuffed the skin off his
knees. After I gave her a hug and told her that I didn't blame
her, she hugged me tightly in return and then started sobbing.
I believed that at this facility, the nurse and administrator were
the only people with the authority to make a decision to call
the paramedics. My heart went out to these twentysomething
caregivers who formed deep relationships with their residents
and who obviously felt responsible. I repeated that I didn't fault
her or any of the other caregivers at all. The nurse never came
outside while we stood there.

The firefighters were leaving on their truck, and the paramedics had loaded Lee into the ambulance by the time I left
the distraught caregiver on the sidewalk. One paramedic asked
me a few follow-up questions about my husband's health history and quickly entered the information into his iPad, while
another attended to Lee, hooking up the cardiac monitor and
an IV. When I mentioned Lee's blood-thinner medication and
past heart attacks, that information seemed to add to the paramedics' sense of urgency. They told me that they had found
abrasions on his knees, elbow, and one shoulder.

"He must have hit the floor hard," a paramedic told me.

The ambulance's lights were on but not the siren. I was
able to follow without going too much over the speed limit.
Ten minutes later, we arrived at the closest hospital. As the
back doors of the ambulance opened, I ran up and handed over
the list of medications that I had absentmindedly tucked into
my pocket. Once inside, hospital staff asked for Lee's insurance

cards while he was whisked away for a brain scan. Much sooner than I expected, the attending ER physician came to report that Lee had a serious subdural hematoma, a large pool of blood trapped between his brain and skull. The doctor showed me the brain scan on a screen in the exam room, and it was obvious even to me that the accumulating blood was shoving Lee's brain far over into the right side of his skull.

"Your husband will die if we don't do something quickly," the ER doctor said. "He probably needs surgery to relieve the pressure."

I already knew that pressure in the brain can herniate the brain stem, which would be instantly fatal.

"Will you approve surgery if we determine that's the best solution?" the doctor asked.

What is best for Lee? I have no idea! I asked the doctor to call a family member who worked in the medical field for the decision, but the doctor said no, there wasn't time.

"I need an answer right now, from you," the doctor declared as he moved toward the door.

I replied, "Yes, please do whatever it takes to keep my husband alive."

I believed that was the answer Lee would want me to give, based on the conversations we'd had when we had completed our durable power of attorney for health care forms years ago. At the time, Lee had chosen his preferences for care in life-threatening situations.

"We'd like to administer IV platelets to try to counteract the blood thinner," the doctor said. I nodded my head yes before he rushed away. I figured that Lee would need platelets whether or not he had surgery. I just stood there, frozen in place, wondering if I could be asleep, having a nightmare. I kept picturing Lee's brain scan.

Five minutes later, the doctor came back to inform me that

Lee would need to be transferred to the Level 2 trauma hospital fifteen minutes away, where they performed brain surgeries. It was the same hospital where Lee had his heart surgeries.

The ER doc lowered his voice, I thought to tell me an important piece of news. "I'd like to ask," he started. "What happened between 2:00 a.m., when your husband fell, and now?"

The doctor looked very serious as he waited for my answer, then rolled his eyes just as the medics had when I retold the story in two quick sentences. He followed up to ask me for the name of the facility and its nurse.

Two ER nurses appeared with Lee on a gurney; the transfer ambulance was ready. I signed some form, held Lee's hand until a special transfer nurse appeared, then ran to my car so I could follow the ambulance.

At the second hospital, a neurosurgeon appeared almost immediately and began an examination. The doctor believed from the progress so far that the platelets were going to slow or stop the bleeding, and Lee was quickly moved into a room on the neurology floor. By now it was early afternoon. They gave Lee half of a sandwich, and he was able to eat it, albeit with closed eyes.

A second scan was ordered in the early evening, and the neurosurgeon came back to tell me the good news: the platelets were working. The bleeding had stopped, some of the pooled blood had already been absorbed, and the pressure inside Lee's head was improving.

"It's possible the subdural hematoma will completely resolve naturally if things continue as they have," the doctor said.

I sent up a silent prayer of thanks. Lee was put on steroids to help with the absorption of the blood, and they were going to hold tight and not do the surgery as long as this rate of progress continued. The neurosurgeon took at least ten minutes to explain brain bleeds in general and Lee's condition in particular as he showed me the new scan. Then he asked if I had any questions, which allowed me the ability to share my concern about the past hospital-induced delirium returning.

"Your husband will be medicated to make an episode less likely," he assured me.

Then, to my amazement, this neurologist gave me his personal cell-phone number and told me to call him anytime, day or night, if I felt the need. I felt my shoulders immediately drop, my jaw unclench, and my hands relax at the knowledge that I could reach the doctor.

Lee was asleep more than awake. Even when at his most awake state, he wasn't fully conscious. He could barely form words and badly slurred those he could utter. I went home around midnight and slept well, trusting that he was going to fully recover, knowing that Lee would be medicated well enough to prevent the delirium, and completely convinced that he had a fully competent neurosurgeon. When I returned the next day, it was apparent that the doctors believed Lee's condition would continue to improve without surgery and that he would survive, although it would take time to know if he had suffered any brain damage.

Taylor called me on the second day. She wanted to give me news about an in-depth investigation she had mounted into the situation. It was obvious that she was genuinely upset that Lee's brain bleed had not been treated more quickly. I really appreciated that she took full accountability for her nurse's decision not to call for the paramedics, at the very least once Tanya had seen Lee in person.

"Can I be called from now on after any fall, regardless of whether Lee seems fine or not?" I asked. I passed on to her what the ER doctor had told me: that on the initial CAT scan, there was evidence of another small brain bleed from not long before, which had healed on its own. I remembered that Lee had fallen a few days earlier, when the activities director had taken a group outside for a walk. The staff had also told me at that time that he was fine. I now could see why there is such a strong recommendation to seek medical advice anytime a person on blood thinners has a fall or a blow to his or her head. Taylor put an order in place on Lee's medical record at the facility, and it was always followed from then on.

Forty-eight hours after being admitted to the hospital, Lee regained his speech and kept looking more and more alert. Then, on the fifth day in the hospital, he began to act as though he might have had another brain bleed, slurring his speech and acting groggy. I called the neurosurgeon's cell-phone number and told him about the changes in Lee's condition.

"I'll be right there," he simply said.

While waiting for the doctor, I stood by Lee's bedside, holding his hand, watching the nurse get a round of medications ready. When I recognized one of the drugs by its distinctive pill shape and color and then noticed that she was putting two of that medication into the pill cup, I stopped the nurse before she handed the cup to Lee and told her that he usually took only one. She rechecked the medication orders, then looked mortified but said nothing. We both knew at that moment that Lee's slurred speech probably meant he'd had a double dose of that medication previously and that he likely didn't have a second brain bleed. I called the doctor's cell phone again to tell him the news, so he didn't waste time coming to Lee's room. The doctor immediately submitted discharge paperwork.

Lee had spent several days in the hospital, yet it was the easiest stay ever for him and for me as his caregiver. The neurosurgeon had taken the potential delirium seriously and made sure that Lee received proper medications. He'd checked on Lee twice a day, every day, and had given me all the information there was to give each time. And, after receiving his cell-phone number, I knew I had somewhere to turn if needed.

After four weeks on a steroid medication; regular visits

to McMillan by a physical therapist, occupational therapist, and speech therapist; and monthly rechecks with the neurosurgeon, Lee fully recovered except for dragging one toe as he walked when he was tired. He didn't remember that he had been in the hospital, suffered a brain bleed, or ridden in a paramedics' ambulance. He had dropped twenty-five pounds. Thankfully, Lee's appetite increased once he was back in a familiar place and into his familiar routine. Addie, the head cook, made sure he was getting the foods that he liked and needed, and the nurse ordered a chocolate Ensure after each dinner to augment that meal. Lee quickly regained the weight.

Two months after the subdural hematoma, I got a call at around midnight; Lee had fallen again. The staff checked him over several times and thought he was OK, but the nurse put him on the phone to me. Lee told me that he had been getting out of bed and just slid his rear end down the side of the bed, ending up in a seated position on the floor. I was heartened by the fact that Lee remembered what had happened and was talking normally. Once I told the staff that I wasn't worried if they were comfortable with his condition, they calmed down and said they would call again if there was any problem. I felt bad for these night-shift caregivers, who seemed to have been traumatized by Lee's prior accident. The following month, Lee had another fall that was much scarier. A brain scan found that he wasn't injured.

I'd heard many times from Jerri and more recently from the staff at McMillan that dementia patients are prone to falls due to problems with balance and strength. They also can't navigate very well around hazards. But I had never grasped the extent of that weakness. I now realized that falls were most likely going to be an ongoing issue for Lee, as they were for many of the husbands of my support-group members. I started carrying a one-page summary of Lee's health history and a medications list in my purse.

THE IDEAL ABSENCE

One month after the brain bleed, I made plans to go to Denver so I could spend Thanksgiving with my younger daughter, son-in-law, and eleven-month-old baby grandson. I'd only seen this youngest grandbaby for two days when he was two months old, after my daughter and son-in-law made a quick trip home. I was dying to spend time with little Finnley.

My flights were arranged so that I would only miss one day's visit with Lee. On Wednesday, I stopped by McMillan on the way to the airport and found that Lee wasn't doing well emotionally. Taylor assured me that he would be fine and that Christine, a truly gifted lead caregiver, was working the entire weekend. She planned to keep an extra eye on him. Just before I left for the airport, Christine came over and told Lee that I was going on a trip to see my new grandbaby. I showed him a picture of Finnley on my phone.

"I'll be the substitute while your wife is gone," Christine said. "If you have any complaint or need anything, you just need to let me know."

Lee smiled. He trusted Christine, and I knew her word was good.

"I'm excited for you to see the baby," he told me. Lee had always adored young children.

I returned on Friday and went straight from the airport to McMillan. Dinnertime had just ended, and Lee was in the living room. As soon as he spotted me walking into the entry, he smiled big. After a bear hug and a kiss, Lee told me he was so glad I was back and asked about the grandbaby. It was obvious that Christine had reminded Lee often where I was. Then he told me that he had a new woman and smiled in Christine's direction. She had no idea how grateful I was for the attention she had given to Lee. I was near tears in gratitude for her and the other caregivers, for Krystal, who had decorated and created Thanksgiving Day activities for the residents, and for Addie, who had prepared turkey, stuffing, mashed potatoes, green beans, and pumpkin pie for the residents' Thanksgiving dinner. Because of these giving, loving women, Lee and I picked right back up where we left off. There were no ramifications at all from the trip to see my baby grandson.

FREEDOM TO BE ILL

Lee needed a follow-up visit every month for three months with his neurosurgeon after having the subdural hematoma. While sitting in the waiting room before the final recheck, I felt like a ton of bricks all of a sudden fell on me. I could barely keep my eyes open. I'd never come down sick like that, so quickly and with such an overwhelming effect. I knew I couldn't leave Lee alone at the appointment, but I didn't want to expose him, the office staff, or the doctor to whatever illness was coming on. Years before wearing face masks would become commonplace, I asked the receptionist for one, and, luckily, she had a box at the ready.

The neurosurgeon gave us good news: Lee's latest scan showed that the hematoma was completely resolved and that he didn't need any more follow-up visits. After helping Lee into our car, I stood outside the passenger door and took a chance, calling one of the family members who didn't work outside the home, hoping she'd be available.

"Can you please come right now to pick up your dad from in front of the doctor's office?" I asked. "I think I'm coming down with the flu and don't want to risk exposing him or taking the illness into the facility."

Lee's older daughter must have already been out and about in that area of town, because it wasn't long before she appeared.

"Hey, Dad, want to go to lunch with me?" she asked.

He was excited to unexpectedly see her and was easily transferred into her car.

I stayed home for three days with the flu. When Lee got upset over not seeing me, one of the caregivers would help him to call, and he could hear from my voice that I was genuinely ill. I was surprised and touched that he had empathy in his voice when he told me that he missed me.

During those three days, Lee did fine. It was clear to me that he felt secure now at McMillan and that he was receiving the services and attention he needed. For the first time in years, I was allowed to properly care for myself. I was free to be sick, to lie under a blanket, and to sleep without any concerns. It felt so weird, that freedom to be ill. I was so grateful I'd found McMillan.

CHAPTER 8

2017

The transition period had been difficult for both Lee and me, but after daily visits for four months, it almost felt like I was entering another version of home when I walked into Lee's room. And he could see that I was not going to abandon him at the facility. We still went out to breakfast, brunch, or lunch multiple times every week. Over time, Lee became secure and comfortable under the routine of McMillan and relaxed in his room. He spent time with Mich every day, too. I was so grateful to Jerri and my support group for encouraging me to find McMillan. It was the answer to my prayers.

By 2017, it was obvious that Lee was in the later stages of Alzheimer's disease. My role now was to help keep him as relaxed, comfortable, and happy as possible. On the days when I saw him smile, when he experienced at least a few moments of joy, it felt like my new purpose in life was being fulfilled.

TIAS

By the beginning of the eighth year after the diagnosis, Lee would occasionally have a short period when he'd have trouble focusing, speaking, and walking, or when he'd become dizzy and very confused. Becky told me that these short episodes he was experiencing were signs of transient ischemic attacks, also known as TIAs or mini-strokes. When the topic came up in a support-group meeting, we found that many of the husbands had TIAs. The bad news: nothing could be done to prevent TIAs. The good news: a TIA episode would seem to end after a few days without any intervention, and most, if not all, of the symptoms would reverse until the next episode.

A HUGE LOSS

Lee never stopped craving going out to brunch and always insisted that we go to the same restaurant every day. It seemed kind of crazy to me, showing up at the same place almost daily. I had to admit I was a little embarrassed as I walked through the door. Yet I made a conscious effort to put on an act as if I were excited each time to be going to the Griddle with Lee, knowing how much he loved it there. When I absolutely needed a break, every four weeks or so, I'd ask and Lee would agree to try a different restaurant for a day. On one particular morning, we went to Joe Momma's.

The hostess seated us in a huge booth, big enough for six diners, which was located at the back of the restaurant. It was a quiet area where there weren't any other patrons, for which I was grateful, because the front of the restaurant was fairly crowded and a little noisy. We had just ordered when Lee got up from the table and started walking toward the front of the restaurant. I noticed that he was pushing himself to walk as fast as possible through the restaurant, a bad sign. For ten minutes, I waited and hoped, then eventually walked up to the front counter and asked the hostess-owner for advice.

"My husband with Alzheimer's is in the men's room and has been in there for quite a while. I think he may need help."

"You'd better go in and check on him," she retorted.

I felt frozen in my tracks and asked, "What if another man walks in?"

"Tell him to get the hell out!" the confident gray-haired owner snapped.

It had become second nature for me to size up people who worked in restaurants, guessing whether I could call on them for help if things went south with Lee. Over the last year, I'd taken note of this middle-aged woman as she built her business to the point where it was really successful now. She was a "take-charge" lady, directing her son and daughter-in-law as they jockeyed crowds on Sunday mornings. I had thought she was someone I could go to if ever I needed help, and her directive this morning gave me the walking papers and the push I needed.

Knocking on the door of the men's room, then opening the door a crack, I called, "Lee, you doing OK? Are you alone in there?"

"I'm in a mess in here," he replied. My heart sank.

Since no one else spoke up from inside the lavatory, I walked in and found Lee sitting in the large stall for disabled patrons. Stepping into the stall, I closed the door behind me, pulled off his shoes and then his jeans, and threw the pants over the top of the side wall. Luck was with us; his jeans and socks were unsoiled.

I had Lee stand up now and hold on to a nearby grab bar as I carefully ripped each side seam of his Depends. Then I quickly grabbed the top back edge and rolled it up from behind his back so that the front section slid between his legs. Once I was done, I laid the rolled up Depends on the floor.

"OK, Lee," I said in a quiet, calm voice, "go ahead and sit back down on the toilet."

Now Lee was sitting there naked from the waist down. I opened the stall door and wet probably thirty paper towels, adding a little soap to them, and then got another thirty or so wet with plain water.

Lee stood up again so I could wash him from his waist down to his midthighs.

"Don't sit down on the dirty toilet seat now," I reminded him as I worked. "Just hold on to the grab bar."

Once he was clean, I dried him with dry paper towels; then he carefully stepped into the jeans as I held them in position. He'd have to go commando. We had been working as fast as possible, wanting to get the heck out of the men's room. I was in a real sweat by that point.

The minute I had his jeans pulled up to his waist, I heard the bathroom door swing open hard and fast with a slam.

"Oh my God," I said under my breath as Lee's eyes widened in panic.

"Can you please give us a few minutes?" I yelled.

"Jesus Christ, why don't you just get a room?" the man yelled back, and slammed the door as he left.

Holy cow!! He thought we were having sex?!

Once I got Lee's sneakers on, I told him to wash his hands carefully and then to wait by the door. He did as instructed. With wads of wet, soapy paper towels, I cleaned up the toilet seat, then threw the Depends and all of the used paper towels into the trash can, pulled out the plastic liner, and tied it off. After I laid the plastic bag by the door, I washed my hands and arms with more soap than I'd ever used in a public bathroom in my life, and we both made a fast exit.

Walking through the restaurant to our booth in the back, I kept my gaze downward toward the floor. I had no idea what the man looked like who had come into the bathroom, and I sure didn't want to lock eyes with anyone in that place. I felt my face burning red all the way back to our booth. As with

most embarrassing situations out in public with Lee, I felt conflicted. Although I had little mental energy left to care what
people thought of us and believed that most people would
recognize the Alzheimer's, there was a part of me that still
cringed, especially when someone assumed we were having
sex in the men's room! Regardless of my emotions, I had to act
normally so that Lee wouldn't feel any worse.

Our breakfasts were waiting on the table, and mine looked
delicious. Even after our bathroom experience, I was still looking forward to the veggie omelet, something blessedly different from the usual fare. Lee would have none of it. He took a
couple bites, then said he wanted to leave. I put my fork down
with a sigh and threw cash on the table.

When we got back to his room, Lee and I made the decision that the breakfast today would be our last restaurant trip
out. I knew that another incident could happen at any time,
and he must have known that, too. I began keeping an emergency backpack with extra Depends, a pair of pants, plastic
grocery bags, and a pack of wipes in the car, just in case they
were needed when we took rides or ran errands.

Lee's doctor and the facility RN and caregivers had warned
me that incontinence was expected in the late stages of dementia. I saw the caregivers take the majority of the residents
at one time or another several times a day to get changed; it
was obvious they were incontinent. One friend had warned
that her husband's incontinence was so bad at night, she had
to use special inserts for his Depends so he didn't wake up in
a huge mess.

Eventually, other bowel-hygiene issues emerged. I discovered a skin infection one day during Lee's shower, the result
of his being unable to wipe completely or forgetting to wipe.
The nurse told me to immediately take him to urgent care,
and they prescribed an antibiotic skin cream to fight the infection. When I reported back to the facility nurse about the

prescription, Becky told me that the caregivers were going to be on a schedule now to use wipes on him several times a day. We knew it would be a fight with Lee, but we also now knew it had to be done.

The facility also put Lee on a new schedule for under-wear changes. They started using adult diapers with little tabs at the sides instead of Depends, so that the caregivers could quickly slip a new pair of underwear through Lee's legs and fasten them at the sides without having to take off his shoes and pants. The whole process took only five minutes or so. But if an accident was extreme, like the one at the restaurant, Lee would have to take a shower, which he absolutely hated and fought. That process could take up to an hour and exhausted him. Luckily, those kinds of accidents didn't happen often.

The professional caregivers at the facility, friends in my support group, and I would exchange tips and tricks, like the rolling technique I'd used in the restaurant men's room. At the same time, we recognized how bizarre it was that this was a normal topic of conversation for us, that we now thought nothing of changing a man's dirty underwear, and that we could even laugh after unusual incidents, like being accused of having sex in a public restroom. Lee soon got used to the routine and even mentioned occasionally that he was grateful for the help.

MOMENTS OF JOY

Once Lee could no longer go out to restaurants, he craved tak-ing rides to see farmland to the west and south of town. Was this because he'd lived on farms during much of his youth and the scenery felt familiar? Every time he felt up to it, we took scouting rides in the county to spot acreages with livestock that were in view from the street. By mid-spring, we had our favorite locations chosen and parked on the sides of the roads to admire newborn foals, calves, sheep, lambs, llamas, and their mothers.

I was a city kid and knew nothing about rural life. Lee was thrilled to teach me about the changes he saw over time in the fields and the animals. I think he could sense that I became genuinely delighted with these outings, and as a result, each ride became energized, with him chatting freely about his years growing up on a farm. Lee would return to the facility tired, satisfied, and ready to settle into his recliner with a Western show on TV. We went on these outings every chance we could get.

The rides in the country brought Lee such joy, it urged me on to find more opportunities for fun. One day, I drove him to his best friend's house so he and Bill could sit on the back deck together, joking and laughing like old times. The next week, I drove Lee out to the dam east of town to see the spring run-off rush out of its gates, forming "rooster tails." We sometimes stopped by a bakery so he could choose his favorite pastries and enjoy them while we took a drive. If he had no energy and was unable to get out, I delivered a TCBY sundae to his room. On the last day of April 2017, we took a chance and violated our decision about restaurants. One at a time, I helped Lee and Mich out of the car, onto the sidewalk, and up to their waiting walkers, then into a little café. Going there was now at the outer edge of both men's abilities, but that lunch really perked up their spirits and was well worth the effort and the risk.

Nearly every Thursday afternoon, Krystal, the activities director, and some of the facility caregivers loaded up a large van to take a group of the most functional residents out for a ride. She might go through a drive-in to get them all ice-cream cones or drive downtown so they could see the Capitol through the van windows. Most of these residents were never taken out of the facility by family and got extremely excited for these weekly trips with Krystal. Lee went a few times but hated riding in the van; he said it was embarrassing being out with a bunch of old people! (He obviously thought he was much younger than he actually was, a common dementia trait.) On the other hand, Mich loved the van rides and went along gladly. I discovered after a few weeks that he always sat next to one lady in particular. It was especially heartwarming to glance through the window and see Mich flirting with his lady friend as the van pulled away from the curb. I always thought that Krystal was brave and kind to bring these wonderful moments of joy to the residents.

A PERFECT STORM

Lee had been dragging his right toe ever since the brain bleed, especially when he was tired. The home-health physical therapist had worked endlessly with him on this problem, and the facility staff and I constantly reminded Lee to lift his toes as he walked. By two months after his release from the hospital, Lee felt finished with his recovery and didn't like hearing the reminders.

Nearly every day since Lee's return to McMillan, Lee and Mich got up and dressed early, well before the 8:00 a.m. breakfast. The two friends would meet at their designated table for a first-thing-in-the-morning cup of coffee, and both told me how much they enjoyed their early-morning one-on-one social time. On one day in particular, they met in the living room and happily chatted while walking together into the dining room. As Addie was putting homemade cinnamon buns into a baking pan, she happened to glance up and saw Lee dragging the right toe on the floor. Before she could say anything, that right toe of his shoe got caught in the cuff of his left pant leg, his legs got tangled up, his body lurched forward, and Lee fell hard on the floor, with his left side taking the full brunt of the impact. Addie and two caregivers rushed to complete the facility's checklist, which included taking his vital signs and checking for pain. Lee's left hip was hurting badly, and he was unable to move his left leg at all. In fact, Addie noticed that it was lying at a weird angle on the floor.

The nurse called 911 while a caregiver called me, and I arrived at the facility just as the paramedics were loading Lee into the ambulance. He was talking loudly to the paramedics, objecting to a trip to the hospital, telling them that he was worried that I wouldn't be going with him. The paramedics and I assured him that I was there now and would drive right behind the ambulance. Although we explained I'd meet him at the hospital, Lee kept protesting loudly until a paramedic decided to help me into the ambulance's front passenger seat so that Lee could talk with me as he rode to the hospital. He had broken his right hip almost sixteen years earlier. I knew what was to come if his left hip was now broken.

The pain was managed well from the start, the nurses knew about the past delirium, and Lee was immobile, so I felt comfortable getting a cab home that evening. But when I arrived at his hospital room early on the second day, the nurses told me that Lee had tried to get out of bed during the night, had pulled out his IV, and was "the biggest handful they'd ever had on a night shift." Now he was refusing to take his medications. While handing a pill cup to me, Lee's nurse asked if I could give it a try. He did take the medications one at a time from me, swallowing each one down with some water after a little coaxing. Once done, the nurse immediately asked if I could arrive as early as possible, ideally by 7:00 a.m., and stay as late as possible, until around 10:00 p.m., so that I could give Lee all of his medications.

"He's much calmer when you're around," she added.

It was easy getting into a hospital routine—trying to

convince Lee to use a urinal, encouraging him to eat meals and snacks, cheering on his physical therapy, helping the nurses scoot his body up in bed, reading to him, tuning in to his favorite TV shows, and mostly just plain entertaining him. I had brought a book along to read during downtimes but never had any.

By the third day, it dawned on me just how extraordinarily busy the orthopedic nurses were on this floor. They were never at the nurses' station and constantly ran up and down the halls. The sounds coming from some of the nearby patients' rooms led me to wonder if most of the other patients had dementia, too. When Lee's nurse came by to check on him on that third day, I asked.

She pushed a strand of hair out of her face and said, "If you can believe it, every single one of the patients on this floor either came in with a dementia diagnosis or has had a diagnosis post-surgery."

The nurses were being overwhelmed by this dementia perfect storm. Now that I was aware of the situation, I could overhear that many of the families were struggling. It came to me that I'd read and had been told by Becky that anesthesia or surgery often brought about a completely unexpected dementia diagnosis for some seniors. Surgery really affected those who already had a dementia diagnosis, too. I felt so bad for everyone involved on the ortho floor.

After that terrible first night, the nurses tried to reserve a hospital sitter for Lee for the night shift, but none were available. They asked me to try, too, and I was also unsuccessful. To be honest, I didn't think that outside sitters would help anyway—Lee probably wouldn't tolerate having a stranger in his room. I found out a few months later, when reading his hospital insurance record, that the hospital had resorted to using a strong drug to keep Lee calm at night. But thank goodness, that was the worst of it. He never had what I would define as severe agitation when I was with him during this hospital stay. I wondered if this good luck was due to the choice of medications or if he understood that he had no choice but to lie in bed.

REHAB

Arrangements were made for Lee to be under a rehabilitation facility's care for a while once he was released from the hospital, and Lee's hospital records were passed on to the rehab facility beforehand. Several days before the transfer, the rehab facility called my cell phone and told me that I had to hire day and night sitters for Lee or they would not accept him. Where was I going to find 24/7 sitters for the rehab stay when the agencies had no one available during his hospital stay? I called Jerri in a panic, and she called around her network. One agency owner was willing to fill the request, but only for the daytime hours. The rehab facility agreed to that arrangement.

Physical therapists at the rehab facility were supposed to work with Lee for an hour twice every day. By the middle of the first week, Lee refused to comply. Then he started becoming very anxious every afternoon. Then he began acting out at any time of the day. Only one sitter was able to get him calmed down—by taking him for a ride around the facility in his wheelchair. Being in a strange, stark, hospital-like environment was really throwing Lee. I spent hours every day at the rehab center trying to keep him calm and making sure he participated in physical therapy and complied with the physical therapists' instructions. At the same time, the medical staff added medications to try to manage Lee's agitation. About a week after he was admitted to rehab, one of the physical therapists asked to meet with me.

"Lee is so drugged up now, he really can't participate in the sessions. I tried to rouse him for the morning session today and wasn't successful."

I had noticed Lee's sleepiness but was shocked by the fact that he couldn't do any PT. *What's the point of being in a rehab facility if he can't take part in their therapy sessions?* I wondered. I went to the charge nurse and requested a list of the medications Lee was receiving at the facility; the report was six pages long. Then I requested a meeting with the nursing supervisor. The next day, at the meeting with Lee's older daughter and me, the supervisor agreed to work on arranging a new combination of medications that would allow Lee to be awake enough to do physical therapy, one that would also keep the pain, anxiety, and agitation tamped down to a manageable level.

In the end, the daytime-sitter situation didn't work out. Lee hated having strangers in his room and fought hard against them. And there was the professionalism issue that is far too common with agency caregivers, which caused me to burn through new sitters faster than the agency could find replacements. One sitter monopolized the specialty recliner designed for those who have had hip-replacement surgery; I discovered Lee in pain while sitting in a wheelchair as she sat back in the recliner. Another sitter disappeared for hours at a time; I couldn't find her anywhere. A third made long phone calls, arguing with her family and friends while sitting in the room. I discovered Lee struggling to hear the TV and upset about her yelling into the phone just feet from his ear. I received a complaint from another patient's family, telling me that I needed to do something about a fourth sitter who stood in the hallway visiting loudly with passersby. Even the nurses had become frustrated by some of the sitters, and they ultimately suggested it might be better if I stayed with Lee from 8:00 a.m. to 10:00 p.m. instead, noting that he was calmest when I was with him. I called the sitter agency and ended their service. The situation wasn't surprising. When using agency caregivers at home, I'd needed to fire a few of the sitters sent to our home because these caregivers' hearts were obviously not in the work. Agencies had a really hard time keeping fully staffed due to the low pay and the demands of the job.

The time at rehab was worth the effort. Lee complied with the physical therapy, and the facility's therapists were expert. Lee recovered amazingly well. On March 6, exactly one month after breaking his hip, he returned to McMillan. Everyone welcomed him with big hugs, and Addie had a cake ready for a little celebration. Lee was beyond thrilled to be back in his familiar environment and with his friends. He continued with home-health physical therapy and occupational-therapy sessions at McMillan and recovered so well that, after another month or so, it wasn't apparent at all that he'd recently had hip-replacement surgery.

It was a coincidence that Becky had just reassessed Lee's abilities using an activities of daily living (ADL) checklist right before he broke his hip. The timing gave her the ability to compare a "before" assessment to a new "after" assessment to determine just how much his condition had declined as a result of the surgery, anesthesia, and hospitalization. She told me that she had been working in the geriatrics field for two decades and found that just about all of her senior patients who had surgery suffered scattered declines. Lee did experience some declines, though after a few months, most of his abilities improved to near pre-surgery functionality.

The orthopedic surgeon ordered a different kind of walker for Lee, one that had wheels on the two front legs and little ski caps on the bottoms of the back legs. The PT told me that this kind of walker was much more stable than the kind with four wheels and a seat. During the weeks right after surgery, Lee leaned heavily on the new walker, but after he was completely recovered, he often balked at using a walker at all even though the physical therapists thought he needed it. I had observed other residents either forget to use their walkers or resist using them. The caregivers at McMillan had to literally set the walkers in front of these folks and insist that they use them. Five minutes later, they'd find a resident without his or her walker and have to hunt it down again. Lee became one of those non-compliant walker residents.

TERMINAL RESTLESSNESS

A year after his move into the memory-care facility, Lee slept through my entire visit. In the past, I'd read a book in his room while waiting for Lee to wake up, and he never slept for more than thirty minutes. This time, he never woke up. It broke my heart to hear from the night-shift caregivers that my husband was now tortured by sleep deprivation, spending much of the night sitting on an easy chair in the living room, watching the night shift go about their tasks. The caregivers kept a stack of throws by the fireplace and laid some across Lee's chest and legs as he sat watching them, hoping he'd fall asleep in an easy chair. He chatted with them and only catnapped off and on all night long. After consecutive sleepless nights, he'd look weak and walk with a weird gait, leaning way forward, with his chest almost parallel to the ground, as he propped himself on the walker. He dragged his toes along the carpet, too tired to completely lift his feet. His face looked gaunt, with huge permanent bags under his eyes. Lee took catnaps at the drop of a hat.

I got the idea to go to the facility one evening and lie next to Lee in bed, hoping that he could relax and fall asleep with me there. He had always loved falling asleep next to me. When I tried that now, I could feel his body quivering all over, just as I'd seen happen for years with the tiny muscles between his thumb and pointer finger. These twitches were almost imperceptible, infinitesimal movements that I could feel going on everywhere on his body. Lee wasn't aware of them, but occasionally he would say that he felt like he wanted to jump out of his skin when he tried to go to sleep. I learned that these tiniest of little spasms were a late-stage dementia symptom called terminal restlessness.

Becky was constantly battling sleep issues in her patients. It was an intermittent problem for some, chronic for others. A few completely switched their days and nights, while others, like Lee, barely slept at all, day or night. Becky and the staff tried everything, including sitting by a patient's bedside and lightly rubbing their backs or upper arms. They knew that a chronic lack of sleep could result in falls and other health issues.

Becky told me about a weighted blanket, a type of comforter with weights or magnets sewn inside, which sometimes helped those with terminal restlessness (and those with autism). These blankets can weigh between ten and twenty pounds each and are expensive, over one hundred dollars. I figured it was worth a try and immediately ordered one on Amazon. When it came the next day, the blanket was so heavy, I could barely lift it. I wasn't sure how or why this blanket worked, but Lee often got a three- or four-hour stretch of sleep while under it.

CHAPTER 9

2018

I'm not going to sugarcoat the account of Lee's disease and care during 2018. Most caregivers want and some will need information about what they might expect at the end stage of dementia. But I'm sure a few of the stories will be hard to hear. Please keep in mind that every case of dementia is different. Many of the people struck by dementia have symptoms and behaviors that are nothing like my husband's case.

Every single day of 2018 was a struggle, for Lee, for his nurses, for his facility caregivers, and for me. Lee was so exhausted, he was debilitated. Becky and I were beaten down, too. The difficulty of Lee's Alzheimer's-disease case was in stark contrast to the other cases at McMillan. He was requiring at least double the typical time and attention from the staff and nurses and now needed nearly all of my waking hours. At the start of every day, I wondered if this would be the day that Taylor would tell me Lee had to move out of McMillan. It was an unbelievable blessing that everyone at McMillan continued to work as a team to help Lee.

FRIENDSHIPS

Just minutes after walking into McMillan on move-in day, Lee had been introduced to Mich. During her introductions, Taylor made a special point of the fact that they both had been lifers in the US Air Force. They took to each other immediately, forming a strong relationship right from the start. From the way Lee and Mich talked during the months after meeting, it seemed that the speed of their relationship-building was a product of the USAF veterans' brotherhood.

One afternoon in 2017, the guys were walking down the hall from Lee's room toward the living room when another male resident intercepted Mich. The six-foot-tall man started aggressively bumping into five-foot-seven-inch Mich. Lee had been trailing behind Mich but noticed right away what had happened up ahead in front of him. He grunted loudly, like a weight lifter, as he pushed his walker as fast as he could toward Mich. When he got even with the aggressor, six-foot-two-inch Lee gave a hard shove into the man's side while making that grunt noise again. The guy slammed into the wall and looked shocked.

Lee yelled, "Get the hell out of here!"

A caregiver saw the entire incident from across the living room and ran as fast as she could to get that antagonist into another room. I realized then how much Lee cared about Mich. (The aggressor moved out of McMillan a few days later.)

Mich had adjusted well to McMillan right from the start, enjoying his new life there. So, Taylor asked him to help Lee see the positives of living there. I would occasionally hear Mich point out an aspect of McMillan that he appreciated and noticed that Lee really took his statements to heart. Mich was also an empathetic listener, a good friend, astutely providing very effective interference for Lee's anxiety many times during the first year.

I suspected that Mich didn't have dementia at all. He had amazing insights into life and the world, never forgot anything that he saw or heard, and always seemed well oriented. I came to believe that he was allowed to stay at McMillan as a favor to his family, who also had Mich's sister at McMillan. She definitely needed a memory-care placement. Mich's niece-caregiver, Penny, visited her mother and uncle often. She and I had worked together during the late 1980s and early 1990s and were thrilled to see each other when our paths unexpectedly crossed at McMillan.

On the afternoon of May 22, 2018, Penny sent word to me that Mich's condition had suddenly taken a turn. He was unconscious, and his family was taking turns sitting with him in an around-the-clock vigil. I dropped by to give support to Penny and to say goodbye to Lee's dear friend. It was heartbreaking that Lee couldn't be there. Becky and Taylor had decided that Lee was incapable of dealing with his friend's death, and I agreed.

Just three days later, Lee and I were sitting in the sun on the patio when Mich appeared in a wheelchair! The caregiver who was pushing him said that he had improved quite a bit and was asking to see Lee. I was shocked and elated. Before the caregiver could even walk away, Mich and Lee saw a military plane fly overhead and got super excited. After they had identified the plane model, their conversation evolved into a long storytelling session. Mich was quite a bit older than Lee and had fought in three wars. He took on the role of historian as he opened up to us in a way that I had never heard before, about the wars, about his volunteering for service at seventeen years of age when World War II began, about how he and other young men were immediately assigned as fighter pilots, about the scant training they had received before being sent into their first air battles, and about how frightened he'd been. Lee sat still, mesmerized by Mich's stories.

The conversation and sunshine seemed to really brighten both men's spirits.

After that time on the patio, I saw Mich around McMillan nearly every day—having coffee in the dining room or watching TV in the living room. In fact, he improved to where he could walk on his own with a walker, tiring quickly but otherwise looking like his old self. I heard from Penny that Mich had said that he hadn't been ready to die. He wanted to say goodbye to a few more people, and that was why he had recovered.

As Lee's condition continued to go downhill in 2018, he began to pull away from friends. He rarely had coffee with Mich now and never spent time with him as he had in the past. I was told that this pulling away was a natural process for those near death. By late August, it seemed that Lee had forgotten about Mich's and his admiration for each other and, eventually, even about their friendship. At times, Lee would get very grouchy for no apparent reason, and during one of those episodes, he said some unkind things to Mich. At that point, Taylor decided that we needed to keep Lee and Mich apart, for both of their sakes. I could see that this change was very difficult for Mich, who missed spending time with Lee, even though he told me that he knew Lee's behaviors were a result of the Alzheimer's, not Lee's fault. Mich began to get more tired and took most of his meals in his room.

On September 22, Mich suddenly became bedridden again and died three days later, at the age of ninety-five. By then, Lee had forgotten that he had known Mich. I was very sad about Penny's loss and felt honored to have known Clarence Michaud, a true American hero.

There were other close relationships at McMillan. Two of my favorite ladies walked arm in arm from one area to another and from one activity to another, laughing together and providing support for each other when one became upset. They often swapped outfits and did up each other's hair, almost as if they were high-school besties.

A few married couples came and went, but one couple in particular stood out. Although most of the couples seemed to bicker a lot, this one couple seemed extremely close, sticking by each other's sides every waking minute. A few months after I met them, I found out that this loving couple actually hadn't known each other before moving into McMillan and that they actually weren't married at all. The man and woman took to each other instantly, insisting that they were married and fighting to live in the same room. The caregivers couldn't keep them apart. Taylor called in the families, who decided to allow the couple to live together even though the woman was already married to a healthy man outside of the facility. If this "marriage" made the couple's last days happy, the families felt they had to allow it. The "wife" died a year later.

Two ladies at different times tried to form a couple with Lee. Betty stalked him for weeks, which greatly upset him; he worried that I would think he encouraged her. I had to constantly reassure him that I could tell she was the instigator, until the caregivers miraculously found a way to get her to let go of her obsession over Lee. The second lady sent him into a screaming session. One evening, Lee walked into his room and found her lying naked on his bed! From what I was told, he started screaming, "If my wife walks in here and sees you in my bed, you're going to cause my divorce. Get the hell out of here!!" Caregivers ran in and pulled the lady out of the room before Lee decked her. The lady did the same thing to two more men, telling Taylor that she had sowed wild oats as a teenager and that she wanted to do it now, too. A month or two later, I realized that I hadn't seen her for quite a while; she must have moved out.

MAJOR DECLINE

There were times during the past few years when Lee would spontaneously start a pretend game. While sitting together at breakfast or lunch in a restaurant, he'd begin to "what-if" a vacation to Seville, Spain, or to Oxford, England, or to a cabin in the mountains, or to some other fun destination. Lee would weave an intricate itinerary into a story and talk about all of the characteristics that he loved most about his fantasy destination. We'd both get excited about the idea of traveling again, even though I knew that the trip was impossible. I think Lee knew deep down that we were engaging in a wishful-thinking game, yet he got caught up in it all the same. He would always hug and kiss me when we reached our car after he'd had one of these fantasies, then forget about it by the time we got home.

By the summer of 2018, Lee's Alzheimer's was in my face, undeniably there all of the time. We couldn't play pretend any longer. I held my breath every time I walked into the facility, wondering what I would find. The main areas of this decline—disorientation, fatigue, lack of appetite, swallowing difficulties, hygiene issues, and agitation—became indisputable red flags, warning of the Alzheimer's increasing toll on Lee's mind and body, providing testimony to the fact that the clock was running out.

Disorientation

Lee's disorientation during spring and summer 2018 was never constant, or at least he never let on if it was. His symptoms could be as simple as waking up from a nap and saying things like "My thinking is really bad." At other times, Lee's view of the world around him would shift. For example, on one country drive in early spring 2018, Lee started shouting, "Look out, stop!" I immediately pulled the car over onto the dirt shoulder.

The road was narrow, with a line of really tall power poles forming a left border. I peered at the spot where Lee was fearfully pointing—straight ahead—and all I saw was blacktop. Then I noticed the shadows. A strong western sunlight was hitting the power poles and casting strips of shade horizontally across the roadway. After I asked a couple of questions, it dawned on me that Lee thought these shadow stripes were bodies lying across the road. I needed to diplomatically help Lee see the shadows for what they were.

"Lee, I'm wondering if your cataract surgery has made your eyes see the shadows on the roadway differently? Do you see the power poles over there? That's where the shadows are coming from. The dark stripes across the street are definitely not bodies."

Lee gazed ahead; I could tell he was unconvinced.

"Watch me," I instructed as I got out of the car and walked over to stand between two of the power poles. I pointed at my shadow, which was cast onto the blacktop of the street, then moved a little so he could see that the shadow moved with me. That calmed Lee down, and he allowed me to drive on, although he did stare hard as we passed over each strip of shade.

On another day in May, it came out in conversation that Lee thought he was still on active duty in the Air Force and was worried about what was going to happen to us when he retired. Since telling him that he had retired a long time ago might be traumatizing, I promised that once he decided to retire, his Air Force pension and my state pension would set us up. He seemed upbeat after that.

In mid-May, Lee declared that he was aging quickly, and this thought had him really upset. I suspected that he had looked in a mirror and had been shocked to see how old he looked. As with most advanced-dementia patients, Lee expected to see a face in the mirror that was decades younger.

On the first of June, Lee was sitting in an easy chair in the living room when I arrived after lunch. He seemed happy and started talking about his mother as though she were still alive.

"When did I last talk with her?" he asked.

"You just talked with your mother on Mother's Day. She's doing fine," I fibbed.

After he claimed he remembered the call, Lee's speech became incoherent, and he fell asleep in the chair.

Ten days later, I arrived to find a husband who was happy but who also had concerns about items missing from his room. Two keepsakes he'd picked up when living in Seville, Spain—carved wooden Man of La Mancha figures—were nowhere to be found. Lee went on and on about what the wooden Don Quixote and Sancho Panza meant to him, who might have stolen them, and how upset he was. Caregivers promised that they would keep their eyes open for the items. I looked all around his studio and in the common areas of the facility—no wooden figures. A few days later, as I helped Lee in the bathroom, I noticed that he didn't have any socks on. When I opened his sock drawer to get a pair, I saw a big lump in the back of the drawer, something rolled up in black dress socks. It was the Man of La Mancha figures!

A week later, I noticed that Lee was drooling and could barely walk. After I convinced him to sit in his wheelchair, we moved to the front porch. I was hoping that a breath of fresh air and a view of the sky would help to brighten his spirits. But when I pushed him out onto the porch, Lee thought that the sunlight beaming down on the concrete sidewalk and driveway was snow. It was disturbing him to feel the warmth of the sun yet to see that the snow wasn't melting. We went back inside. The milkshake I'd stashed in his freezer brought smiles, but Lee couldn't figure out how to use the straw. I fed it to him with a spoon.

During lunch in late June, Lee accidentally spilled his coffee on Bill, a resident and tablemate whom he really liked. It was a challenge to follow what Lee was saying, since he was using random words and partial sentences, but I got the gist of it. He was mortified. I assured him that Bill would forgive him.

Near the end of June 2018, Lee was waiting for me by the front door and looking confused when I arrived. Caregivers had been trying to get a urine specimen, which they routinely did for all residents. The collection pan that was situated between the toilet base and toilet seat scared Lee. After half an hour of explanations, he sat down and gave me a specimen, but he was still scared of that contraption.

During the second half of 2018, I became less shocked by the disorientation, but it still broke my heart to see my brilliant husband losing touch with reality.

Fatigue

To me, Alzheimer's disease is synonymous with fatigue. Everyone I knew with the disease suffered from severe fatigue. And Lee's sleep apnea just exacerbated the situation. I didn't think the fatigue could get any worse until early May 2018, when, for the first time, Lee said that he wasn't up to a ride. For years, he had pushed himself through pain and all sorts of illnesses just to cruise along the roads in the hills. The fatigue had to have been overwhelming for him to say he wasn't up to going out.

Then, on May 23, the director, the nurse, and the lead caregivers decided that Lee shouldn't go out for rides at all. While Taylor was explaining her decision to Lee, Sam, a lead caregiver, took me aside to explain that Lee was so exhausted and weak after our most recent rides, they worried that he would have a heart attack. He usually fell right to sleep for a nap once we got back to McMillan after the rides, so I hadn't realized their complete effect.

On June 7, Becky called in the morning to let me know that

both she and Taylor believed that Lee would never stop being upset about missing his rides. Not going out had been causing him to descend into fits of agitation. It was a dilemma—the outings were becoming too much physically for Lee, but missing them was too much emotionally. They recommended taking Lee out for a short ride today, and if it went well, to take him for short rides on Mondays and Wednesdays from now on.

As we drove the short distance to TCBY, Lee mumbled incomprehensibly. After I navigated the car through the drive-through, Lee couldn't manage to hold his ice-cream dish. I parked the car so I could hold the container for him, but Lee also couldn't figure out how to use the spoon. It felt so very strange to be sitting there in front of the store feeding the frozen yogurt to Lee, and so tragic that his condition was to the point that this formerly super-capable man couldn't even feed himself. We immediately returned to the facility, and Lee went right to sleep in the recliner. After hearing about today's ride, Becky confirmed the new Monday-and-Wednesday schedule. It was a relief. Instead of having to say flatly that we were unable to take rides, now when Lee lobbied hard to go out, I could remind him of the outing schedule and count down the days till the next ride. I hoped he could live with that—and that the rides weren't too much for him.

At the beginning of June, the cook let me know that Lee was too weak to hold his coffee mug and dropped it every day now, spilling coffee on himself and others. I ran by Starbucks and found the perfect coffee mug with an attached top that wouldn't spill if dropped. Eventually, Lee didn't even have the strength to hold that cup and couldn't remember how to drink out of its flip-top anyway. The facility staff and I never could think of an effective solution for the spills.

By mid-June, Lee sometimes didn't even have the strength to open his eyes, talking to me with his eyes shut. He started having difficulty standing, even when using a walker. I left immediately when he was that tired, putting him to bed and hoping he'd sleep if I wasn't there.

Eating and Swallowing

On June 19, Becky called me in the early evening to tell me about a medication change, and the news made me panic.

"What if he's taking too many meds already?" I asked. "Lee has been drooling. Doesn't that mean he is already overmedicated?"

Becky patiently explained that the current medications were very typical for senior, late-stage dementia patients and were at the standard recommended dosages. If Lee was drooling, it was likely a sign that he was losing his ability to swallow. My heart sank.

I was scared to death of the swallowing difficulties that sometimes come with late Alzheimer's disease. My father had contracted aspiration pneumonia eight years earlier, from choking on food particles and breathing them into his lungs. Two days before he died, he kicked and fought in a panic, feeling as if he were drowning on his own infected mucus that had built up in his lungs and throat. After he passed, I prayed to God that no one else I knew would ever have to suffer that kind of death.

Becky informed me that as soon as we ended our call, she would put Lee on a special soft-foods diet and instruct the med techs to crush and mix his medications in applesauce. The caregivers were on duty in the dining room during mealtimes, keeping an eye out for residents' choking. Yet memory-care facilities don't have the manpower or a mandate to individually feed residents. From then on, I tried to be with Lee during lunches and dinners as often as possible, since the more tired he became, the more his risk of choking increased.

At the end of June, Addie told me it was a good thing I

was bringing Lee ice cream most days because his appetite had dropped dramatically. She had to coax him to eat breakfast, which had always been his favorite meal, and now he barely ate lunch or dinner. Lee was beginning to lose weight, a bad sign for those with late-stage Alzheimer's.

Hygiene

By spring of 2018, Lee needed help with all aspects of hygiene. Once I noticed some nicks and cuts on his face, I realized he couldn't shave himself. I found a great electric razor at Costco that worked on both wet, lathered skin and dry skin. Lee loved sitting back in his recliner while I shaved him and always joked about having a private valet.

He also didn't seem to mind McMillan caregivers' involvement in the bathroom anymore. Lee was completely incontinent now, so he needed help changing his underwear many times a day. The facility caregivers and I approached that chore as a team. They recorded his underwear changes in their patient notes. When I did it, I used a Sharpie to record the date and time on the back of his incontinence underwear, so the caregivers could easily see when it had been changed by me.

By the end of June, one of Lee's most frequent conversation topics was how much he hated incontinence underwear. Then one day, I went to undress him for a shower and discovered that he was going commando! When I asked lead caregiver Laura if she knew what was going on, she followed me back into Lee's bathroom. We found his underwear shredded and buried in his trash can. For some unknown reason, he had shredded the stuffing from the lining, making it look like a pile of snow in his trash can. Now I realized that Lee's "I hate diapers" conversations had been a warning that he wasn't going to tolerate the incontinence underwear much longer. This first rebellion was the start of a struggle that went on until the week before he passed away.

The facility staff tried to take over showering at this point, multiple times, worried that the job was getting to be too much for me, but Lee absolutely would not allow it. While he had quit fighting the caregivers' help with toileting tasks and changing in and out of pajamas and clothes, he said it wasn't right for young women to see him completely nude in the shower. After a couple of weeks, the caregivers gave up trying to take over the showering task.

The staff was right; showering had become much more difficult because of Lee's unsteadiness and fatigue. The staff's warnings were taken to heart. Lee needed help with everything to do with a shower now, including undressing. It was safest and easiest for us if he sat on the toilet as I pulled off his clothing. He didn't object when I put a gait belt around his naked chest so that I had something to hold on to as he walked across the bathroom and sat down on the shower chair. The fact that he had trouble retaining body heat and shivered through the entire shower made him even more unstable.

After a shower, I leaned Lee against his bed while I helped to dress him so that he had a soft landing if he lost his balance. The entire twice-weekly process took thirty to forty-five minutes, and by its end, Lee was completely drained, crumpling into his recliner. Wrapped in a throw blanket, he immediately fell asleep.

When I arrived at McMillan on July 6, Lee was in the bathroom, and he stayed in there for quite a while.

"Can I help you, honey?" I eventually asked through the door.

This time, it took a shower to address his incontinence issues and some Mr. Clean (which I kept hidden in a low cabinet) to get the bathroom back in working order. Once he was clean and dressed, Lee thanked me profusely, which broke my heart.

During the second week of July, I found Lee asleep in his recliner with no shoes or pants on. The lead caregiver, Laura, told me it was a sign that his underwear needed to be changed. He could no longer recognize or verbalize what he needed. Since sleep was the number one priority for Lee, the caregivers had been waiting for him to wake up before changing him.

Lee had his winter coat on and was waiting for me when I arrived on July 2. The temperature outside was in the nineties. It took some diplomacy, but he didn't seem to mind changing into summer-weight clothing. While Lee never went on outings anymore, he needed a haircut and was doing relatively well on that day. Taylor and the lead caregiver gave me their approval for a quick trip to the barbershop. The July haircut turned out to be a real challenge, especially as Dewey and I helped Lee up into the barber's chair. It became instantly apparent that this haircut would be his last at Dewey's, as Lee quickly fell asleep sitting up in the barber's chair. It seemed that Dewey knew it, too, as he sadly and quietly cut Lee's hair that last time.

Agitation

If someone were to ask which Alzheimer's-disease symptom was the most impactful on my husband and on his caregivers, anyone who had cared for him for a significant length of time would certainly answer: agitation. By May, Lee's agitation appeared almost daily, and the periods became more and more difficult to manage. It was common for me to arrive at McMillan and find Becky working with him in his room or in the living room, trying to calm Lee before he lost control. She spent untold nights sitting by his bed, trying to help him relax as much as possible. Becky even resorted to keeping an extra set of clothing in her office for those times when she never made it home at night. She consulted with Lee's medical providers and called in psychiatric nurses, all in an effort to find help for Lee. They tried everything, even stopping the two Alzheimer's drugs he'd taken for years. In later stages and in some rare cases, these common drugs were believed to suddenly interact with other drugs in unexpected ways. Nothing helped.

On May 9, as I walked through McMillan's front door, I saw Lee standing in the living room, holding tightly to his walker, with his arms flexed rigidly. The director, the nurse, and two caregivers were all standing equidistant from each other in a semicircle around him, listening to some argument Lee was giving. I knew that this high-level attention meant that he was having a severe episode of agitation. And I assumed, from the way they had positioned themselves, that the staff had fanned out around Lee to protect the other residents in case he might try to throw something.

I walked in purposefully so Lee could see me and said, "Hello," hoping to break his focus on whatever had upset him. Lee turned his gaze from Taylor and acknowledged me. So, I approached, saying something upbeat to see if I could help pull Lee out of this situation by distracting him. When Lee reached out, I thought it was to hold my hand, but instead he unexpectedly grabbed my wrist and squeezed, hanging on with all his might.

"You're hurting me," I said as I winced; he immediately let go.

I could see the concern on Taylor's face—this was the first time she'd seen Lee grab someone while at McMillan. Before the agitation could build (and before I could hear Taylor say the words I'd been dreading: that she would have to expel him from the facility), I quickly took Lee out of the building.

He was excited to get out and calmed down as soon as we

drove toward TCBY. By the time we returned to McMillan, he had forgotten about whatever had triggered the earlier episode. Lee was able to relax in his recliner, although his left arm and leg twitched badly. The morning had been hard on the caregivers, the nurse, and the administrator. I stayed with Lee until past bedtime to keep him occupied and, hopefully, calm. It worked that evening.

On May 31, Taylor decided to try reducing my visits to every other day, hoping that fewer visits would help with his fatigue, which in turn might help the agitation.

"Let's see how he responds to visits every other day for a few days, and then we can go from there," she said.

Becky called me at around 6:00 p.m. on the first day I didn't visit. Lee's condition had degraded into delirium. He'd thrown his walker and other items across the living room, and it took ninety minutes to get him calmed down.

"Lee's agitation was the worst I've ever seen, in anyone, during my two decades of working with dementia patients," Becky told me.

She was going to talk with Taylor about reinstituting our daily rides, Becky said. I could tell by her tone of voice that Lee's situation was nearing the end of the line for McMillan. She was completely exhausted.

On June 4, Lee was very happy when he saw the TCBY in my hand as I walked through the door. In fact, he seemed happy for the entire visit, but that mood evaporated when I got up to leave. I was floored when he accused me of having an affair.

"You're leaving to meet your new lover, aren't you?" he shouted.

Several of my caregiver friends had warned that they'd seen this same type of paranoia in their loved ones, so I wasn't completely unprepared. I have to admit, though, that my heart was crushed by the accusation.

The next day was a skip-a-visit day, and lead caregiver Christine called that evening to tell me that Lee had been extremely agitated for most of the afternoon. She asked if I could come to visit. Lee looked happy when I appeared, but I quickly realized it was because he thought I was taking him out. As soon as he started showing signs of agitation, I left so the situation wouldn't escalate.

That evening, lead caregiver Christine called to let me know that Lee was extremely agitated again.

"I don't think you should come in," she said, "but will you talk with him on the phone?" I did what I could over the phone to calm him down.

By mid-June, everyone involved in Lee's care was worn out. I kept thinking about Jerri's encouragement two years before to move Lee into a facility; "Thank God" became my silent mantra. If caring for Lee was this difficult for multiple people, I knew that I never could have survived these months on my own.

DOWNWARD SPIRAL

When I walked into Lee's room in mid-June, I found him slumped in his recliner, slurring his speech, drooling, and acting confused. I literally ran to the nurses' office.

"I think Lee's had a stroke or another brain bleed!" I told Becky.

She ran at her top speed to Lee's room, checked his vital signs, and examined him.

"I don't think Lee is having a stroke or a brain bleed," she said quietly once she was finished.

Becky had seen it all when it came to dementia and gerontology. I trusted her opinion when she told me that Lee's condition was in a major decline.

Once she finished her explanations, Becky hugged me. I really don't know how it was possible that, with all that was going on in the facility, she was able to stop everything she was doing at the drop of a hat and behave as if nothing else but my husband mattered at that moment, but she did. I realized then how much I had been leaning on Becky almost every day. Her support and hug at just the right time helped me immensely.

The symptoms eased up the next day, yet two weeks later, Becky told me that Lee's condition was worsening further. Although he did still have good days, there were other days when he spoke using only a string of words. When this happened, if I mentally filled in the gaps, I could figure out what he was trying to say. At other times, he might mumble random words, and I had no idea what he was trying to tell me. On really bad days, Lee might see things that weren't there, choke on his saliva, feel lost in familiar places, or be too tired to walk. He stopped noticing that we weren't going out for rides, so our outings ended altogether.

In early July, Becky dropped by Lee's room to ask me to visit her office before I went home. She rarely asked me to meet with her in a formal way. After an hour, I walked back to the nurses' office, where Becky and Logan, the LPN, were working on orders and files. They ushered me in and got right to the point. Becky listed off the significant changes they had recently noticed, and Logan chimed in. I had already noticed all of the symptoms and behaviors they mentioned, so nothing they said was shocking.

Then Becky broke the news: "The home-health nurse practitioner will examine Lee tomorrow to determine if he is qualified for hospice care. That would bring in more resources and support."

To be honest, the referral wasn't a surprise, but the word "hospice" sent a shock wave through me regardless. It was one thing to know in my head that Lee was near the end; it was another thing to hear a medical provider state it as fact. After hearing about hospice from many of my caregiver friends, I knew that this meant there was little time left.

Becky had been routinely sitting up nearly all night at least once a week with Lee, and I could tell by the fatigue written on her face that she desperately needed help. The caregivers were overwhelmed with caring for Lee, too, due to his sleeplessness and episodes of agitation. A couple of months before, Taylor had told me that Lee's care needs were drawing an inordinate amount of attention from the other residents' care and that it wasn't fair to them. She had already upped the monthly fees to the maximum of $9,500 per month to schedule more help. And I had upped the amount of time I was spending at McMillan. I worried constantly that Lee was going to be transferred to a skilled-nursing facility. So, of course, I told Becky I was supportive of a hospice agency's involvement in Lee's care. Besides, I'd heard nothing but good about hospice care from my friends.

Two days later, Becky summoned me back to her office again, and I immediately noticed a very concerned look on her face. The home-health nurse practitioner had determined in her examination that Lee's language abilities were too good to qualify for hospice under Medicare's requirements. I was shocked but said nothing. Then Becky gave me a look, and I could tell she was thinking what I was thinking—that if that nurse had visited three days in a row, at different times of the day, boy would she have come away with a different picture.

Then Becky gave me a stark warning: with her decades-long nursing experience in gerontology, she could tell that Lee's body was shutting down.

"He's reduced his food intake, a sign that his metabolism has slowed," she said. "People can go on for a while in this state, but it's rare."

It immediately struck me that Lee had eaten only half of

his ice cream during our visit today. That had never happened before. Becky stood up and gave me a hug.

"I'm so sorry. Please don't let this denial of hospice care give you a false sense of optimism. Lee's language ability at the one moment in time when he was examined may have disqualified him for hospice, but we know that in many other ways he definitely meets the criteria, and I think he will qualify soon."

Then she said the words I had been anticipating and dreading: "I don't want you be shocked if Lee unexpectedly passes away."

I stayed with my husband through dinner and well into the evening. He was happy to have me there, and I couldn't make myself leave. I thought of John, a resident who'd lived at the facility the first year Lee was there. He looked healthy enough, walked fine, and was a cranky old coot. One midafternoon, he yelled at a caregiver to be quiet so he could hear the living-room TV, then fell asleep in an easy chair as he watched, which was par for the course for John. He didn't wake up, though, when a caregiver tried to roust him for dinner. At the time, I voiced shock at his passing that way. John had talked with me just the day before and seemed with it. Becky explained to me at the time that she had already warned his family; she had seen the signs. Today, Becky was telling me that she was now seeing the signs in Lee. I knew from experience that I needed to trust her judgment. I made an appointment with our clergyman.

A few days later, Lee met my arrival with a big hug. It felt so good to have his arms around me and to see him smiling. Soon after, he fell asleep in his recliner and didn't wake up during the two hours I sat in his room. Becky told me as I was leaving that she had requested another exam for hospice-care eligibility.

After dinner, Lee had a caregiver call to ask me to come back. We sat together, holding hands and watching television until 7:00 p.m., when I helped him into pajamas and eventually tucked him into bed. While lying there with his eyes closed, Lee told me how much he loved me. I closed my eyes and held on to those words for as long as I could, knowing that I wasn't going to hear them much longer. *Could Lee be sensing that his body is failing?* It was getting harder and harder for me to walk out of McMillan.

Lee was very happy to see me the next day. We had lunch together and spent the afternoon on the patio, cherishing his awake time. As I was leaving, Lee's home-health nurse practitioner summoned me as she left another resident's room. She wanted to give me a heads-up that Lee's medication dosages were all being reduced. *Oh my gosh, a time bomb has just been set to go off!*

Becky called the next morning, on July 11, explaining that the nurse practitioner had reduced most of Lee's drugs by half yesterday. Becky couldn't see me clench my teeth, bracing for what was to come.

"Lee was really agitated last night," Becky went on. "I sat with him for nearly two hours to help him calm down."

At 1:15 a.m. the following morning, the staff called to tell me that Lee had fallen out of bed, but they believed he was OK. Later that morning, Becky came by Lee's room, where I was waiting for him to wake up. She led me out into the hall to tell me that, since he was just as sleepy with the reduced medication dosages as he had been before, they could now isolate the cause of the sleepiness and know definitively that it was caused by the Alzheimer's, not his former medication dosages. I had suspected that all along.

But then there was no agitation from July 12 to July 15, four days in a row! I wondered, *Was it some reduced or discontinued drug that was the culprit, causing his former anxiety? Will the drop in agitation be long-lasting?* Lee and I spent the afternoon together on July 15, and he wasn't upset when I left. It was such a relief!

The next day, the anxiety returned with a vengeance. Lee was in the living room, attentively pacing as he watched for me to arrive.

"What town are we in?" he demanded.

From the things he said, it sounded like he thought I had been moving us around, like we were homeless or on the lam and that we were getting ready to move again. Then the agitation gained steam. After a few minutes, Lee picked up his walker and threw it at me. It hit the floor with a crash, and the loud noise shocked him and the other residents. Becky quickly administered a half dose of antianxiety medication, but the agitation kept building, along with the fidgeting of terminal restlessness. I made him a promise that I was not going to leave, that I would be there with him all day and night. And I did anything else I could think of to help calm him, worried that he was going to be expelled from McMillan. He didn't act out again for the rest of the day and night.

Later the next afternoon, a hospice nurse, Amy, who was there to see her patients at the facility, introduced herself and told me that a meeting about hospice was scheduled for the next afternoon. She said she'd call later with more information. I wondered, *Did the nurse practitioner just approve Lee for hospice?* Amy never called, so I called her agency the next morning and learned that the meeting was to be in two days.

On July 18, Lee and I went for a ride to TCBY, which thrilled him even though he wasn't sure where he was. Once back in his room, I turned the TV to his favorite Westerns channel, then walked down to the nurses' office for the meeting about hospice services. Becky, LPN Logan, hospice nurse Amy, and the manager of her hospice agency were there, along with two members of Lee's family who had expertise in health care. It was decided at that meeting that Lee's medical care would be transferred to the hospice agency.

CHAPTER 10

Hospice

Sometime after Lee moved into McMillan, I started wondering but never asked, *Who are these people who just breeze into McMillan like they work there and enter residents' rooms like they are family? What are they doing there? Why doesn't the lead caregiver greet them like she does other visitors?* Eventually, I got the answers to my questions. They were visiting nurses who worked for two types of outside agencies: home-health agencies and hospice agencies.

When residents needed to be in the care of a doctor or physical therapist but weren't up to traveling to the provider's office, their families could contract with outside home-health agencies. These agencies provided visiting nurse practitioners, psychiatric nurses, and physical therapists to homes and facilities in the area. If needed, a home-health nurse practitioner could even call in a mobile X-ray unit. Becky and the LPN, Logan, acted as liaisons between the facility and these agencies and carried out any orders given by their medical-care providers. (If MRIs or CAT scans or other specialized tests or procedures were needed at a hospital, there was a special wheelchair taxi that could pick up a resident and family member.)

Once Lee was too fatigued or weak to travel to a doctor's office, we contracted with a very good home-health agency whose nurse practitioner visited the facility weekly. She worked very well with Becky and seemed to have that same sixth sense about her patients. This home-health NP kept me in the loop after any examinations, but she was difficult, if not impossible, to reach. I still went to Becky if I had questions or concerns.

Once it was suspected that a resident was within six months of death, Becky or the home-health nurse practitioner would inform the family and ask if they would like a referral for hospice care, which provided intensive, end-of-life comfort care. If the family agreed, the resident's physician or home-health nurse practitioner needed to certify that the patient was within six months of death, so that the patient could be qualified for hospice services under Medicare insurance. Once the patient was approved, their family could then contract with a hospice-care agency. Hospice care made specialized equipment available, such as air beds to prevent sores in people who were bedridden. Hospice could also bring in other specialists, too, if needed. Hospice care, including the equipment-rental fees, was completely paid for by Medicare insurance. There were typically four or five residents in Lee's facility at any given time receiving hospice care.

JULY 2018

The fact that my husband was "on hospice" now lay heavy on my heart and mind. Every minute with him felt precious. As I walked into McMillan the morning after the hospice meeting, scanning the living room to see if Lee was there, hoping that we could have a good day together, one of the caregivers mentioned that he had experienced a very, very bad morning. I never knew how to react to this kind of bad news from caregivers about Lee's agitation. I could assume that they were trying to warn me so that I would be extra careful about what I said to him to avoid making the situation worse. Or, knowing that Lee sometimes calmed down with me, maybe they were asking for my help? In most cases, though, my immediate re-action to the news was to feel pity for the staff and Becky and to feel terribly guilty for some unknown reason. I knew how mentally exhausting it was, trying to happen upon some magic phrase or some action that might turn the switch in Lee's head from a state of panic, fear, anger, frustration, and paranoia to a state of somewhat peaceful self-control. I also knew what a time drain the agitation was for the staff and Becky. In the end, I always felt responsible—in a sense, in the way a parent feels responsible for a child acting up in school, perhaps because a demented person couldn't be held accountable for his actions any more than a small child. I was the one who had moved Lee into McMillan and ultimately subjected the caregivers to his agitation. I took on real guilt.

Yet when I stepped into Lee's room that first day on hos-pice, knowing that he'd had a bad morning and expecting the worst, I found Lee happy to see me. Relief hit me like a wave. We held hands and watched TV for hours, and he seemed con-tent. It was a great day until I went to leave. As I moved toward the door, Lee held tight to his walker for balance and walked behind me as fast as he possibly could. The caregivers had to stand between us and block Lee, to give me enough time to enter the door code, open the door, and then push it closed as fast as it would go so it locked again before he got there. It broke my heart to leave that way, to hear Lee shouting after me. He couldn't bear to be separated from me now.

On July 21, Lee was in a good mood when I arrived, but his anxiety grew as time passed. He had some crazy idea that he was making an upcoming move "from this hotel to some-where in Iowa, maybe Sioux Falls" and was worried sick about it. Not knowing where and when he was moving was driving Lee crazy. I tried to convince him that we were not moving, but he refused to believe me.

The next day, I walked into Lee's room and was shocked by what I saw. He was slurring his speech, unable to completely stand on his own, with eyes only open halfway. His face reminded me of the time he'd had a brain bleed. A caregiver helped me get Lee into his wheelchair so that we could go sit on the patio. I was hopeful that being outside would lift his spirits. Although he looked terrible, Lee still had it in him to admire the beautiful cloud formations. He directed me to move his wheelchair every few minutes to get a better view of the clouds. Unbelievably, he stayed outside for two hours watching that sky. Afterward, a caregiver and I helped to get Lee comfortable in his recliner, and then I slipped out of the room as he dozed. As I walked through the living room, I learned from the lead med tech that one of Lee's medications had been increased, which was probably why he was so sleepy. That short aside took a load of worry off my shoulders. If his problem with standing was caused by medication, they would adjust the dosage, and he would be able to stand up on his own by tomorrow. McMillan didn't allow residents to live there if they couldn't support their own weight and help shuffle as they made a transfer from a toilet, shower chair, or bed to a wheelchair. I was always looking over my shoulder, waiting for one reason or another to cause Lee to be moved from the facility. At least today's situation was not it.

Two days later, on July 24, it was almost as if Lee had reverted mentally back to when he had first moved into McMillan. He absolutely did not want to be there and lobbied hard for me to move him out. Thankfully, I was able to redirect him, and after a while he forgot about wanting to leave. I had a doctor's appointment and explained to Lee why I had to shorten my visit. He graciously held my hand and acted sympathetic about my stomach pain as he walked me to the door. After I kissed him goodbye and stepped up to the keypad to unlock the door, he pushed me out of the way and tried to force the door open.

"I'm going to the doctor's appointment with you!" he shouted.

I hung on to the door by the edge of the push bar as Lee shoved hard against it over and over, making a loud clanging noise. I knew that if he kept this up, the door would break. My heart sank for Lee. I could tell that he was terrified for me to leave him that day. *Does he think that I'm so sick that I will die, or go to the hospital, or for some other reason never come back?* I thought. *I never should have told Lee I had a doctor's appointment!* He shoved himself between the door and me and continued pushing as hard as he could on the door's emergency-exit bar.

Amy was in the building and saw what was happening. She came over and told Lee that he had to have a scheduled medication before he could leave, and he immediately stopped fighting with the door. I walked Lee to the lead med tech's wooden lectern so she could give him the medication. That medication had been ordered by the hospice agency's physician when Lee started on hospice. The medication was prescribed by the doctor in such a way so that it could be given when Amy requested it, up to a certain maximum dosage, when these agitation episodes arose.

While he was occupied by the lead caregiver with taking the medication, Amy pulled me aside.

"I'm going to see about getting a pain evaluation for your husband," she informed me.

I sat with Lee for a few minutes, until the caregivers could distract him long enough so that I could run to the door and get it unlocked. Lee sprang up and tried to follow as fast as he could, screaming as I entered the code and then closed the door behind me. I could hear him yelling for me as I walked quickly down the sidewalk. Those cries haunted me for the rest of the day and night. I drove to the doctor's appointment in tears, where I learned that the pain in my gut was diverticulitis. It kept me in bed for two more days until the antibiotic fought back the gut infection.

Lee was cheerful when I arrived back on July 27, a drastic change from three days ago. Whatever medication changes his hospice doctor and nurse had made, they were clearly helping. He talked about the fun we'd had on our trip to Europe in April and May 2000, declaring the vacation the highlight of our lives. I agreed wholeheartedly and was amazed that Lee remembered so many details about a trip we'd taken eighteen years ago and that he was conversing so well. Days like these made my body feel lighter, as if a load had been lifted from my shoulders.

The next day, we sat on the patio and ate sherbet that Addie gave us. Ever since I'd known him, Lee never drank coffee after midmorning. Now, he was reverting back to the old habits of his twenties and thirties, when he had worked shifts as a weatherman and drank coffee regardless of the hour. After he finished a cup of decaf coffee, Lee went to his room and lay back in the recliner. He was half-asleep and content when I left.

July 30 brought hugs and kisses as Lee welcomed me into his room. It brought me back to our first fifteen years together, when he would greet me in the same way when I got home from work. A short drive seemed doable, so we set off for TCBY. During that drive, Lee's mood changed to sadness. A few days earlier, Lee had begun saying that someone had told him that he was going to be stuck in this facility until the day he died and that the only way he would be leaving was in a wooden box. I couldn't believe I was hearing that same ghastly

prediction repeated from his first days at McMillan. The statement had become a sort of mantra over the last few days. I
had no idea how this morbid thought had returned to the front
of his mind. I wondered, *Is he miraculously remembering it
from two years ago? Or did someone recently repeat it to him?
If so, how could anyone purposefully say such a cruel thing to
a person who is under hospice care?* After a few minutes, Lee
stopped repeating the mantra, and I moved on, not having the
mental energy to deal with the issue.

Nurses Amy and Becky both mentioned to me that recent
medication changes had helped; the agitation was much better, day and night. They seemed to feel that they might have
found an answer to getting the agitation under control. I was
hopeful after today's visit.

AUGUST 2018

During the following week, the first week of August, Lee continued to perseverate on the idea that he would be at McMillan
until the day he died and was carried out in a wooden box. It
was unusual for him to remember any fear for long and especially rare for any thought to last for more than a day, let alone
weeks. It was hard on the facility caregivers and me as we
watched him get so upset by such a gruesome thought. From
the day Lee had moved into McMillan, the staff and I had told
him that he was in the facility for rehab. What with his stints
of physical therapy and the hip surgery, this reasoning continued to make sense to him during his two years at McMillan.
Although Lee didn't like the idea of staying at a rehab facility,
it didn't depress him. He always had the hope that he could
improve. But that changed when Lee became caught up in the
thought that he would be at the facility until he died. It was

a devastating shift in outlook, and during the first week of August, he was angry to his core. The macabre thought caused him to lose hope and sleep until, days later, it did eventually fade away.

At the end of the week, Lee complained that his teeth didn't feel right. When I looked in his mouth, I was shocked to see the condition of his lower teeth. They were caked with tartar and yellow goo! There were also two obvious cavities and inflamed gums. My stomach sank from the realization that no one, including me, had thought to look at the areas of his mouth that didn't show when he smiled. Lee sat back in his recliner as if I were going to shave him while I laid a dry towel under his chin and gently brushed his teeth. Every so often, I gave him some water to sip, rinse, and spit into an empty cup. His gums were in bad shape. I had to brush very softly, stopping every few seconds, and then give it up after a minute so his gums wouldn't get sore or bleed. After four days of brushing this way, his teeth and gums looked much better, and he declared that they didn't feel weird anymore. Becky said it was best to let the two cavities go as long as they didn't cause him pain. Dental procedures would have been a nightmare at this point.

When I arrived for a visit one day in early August, I found Lee sitting on the toilet with a pair of incontinence underwear shredded on the floor all around him. He was in a mess, so I had no choice but to strip him while he sat there and put him in the shower. On that day, I had a fleeting thought, a sense, that Lee was losing control over his lower body.

At the end of August, Becky called me at home to let me know that Lee was consistently waking up at 2:00 a.m. They were concerned that his days and nights might be getting mixed up. She asked me to try to keep Lee awake during my visits. I understood the reasoning but had no idea how to do what Becky asked.

OCTOBER 2018

In October, Lee started having vivid nightmares, day and night. A caregiver would occasionally call me to the facility late at night, and on one of those nights, I just couldn't calm Lee down. He was terrified and angry. I kept thinking that there had to be a reason that these super-realistic dreams had just popped up. Eventually, I found out that Lee had been started on a sleep medication on the day the nightmares began. I was beyond frustrated at the situation and with myself. I had forgotten to tell Becky that Lee couldn't take Ambien and texted her right away to request that it be stopped immediately. I had never given input about drugs before, so she knew I probably had a good reason. She could tell that I was dead serious in my request. Within a couple of minutes, I saw the hospice RN, Amy, in the hall as she was leaving another patient and explained to her that Lee had tried the same medication fifteen years earlier with similar side effects. She immediately stopped the drug.

The good news in October: Lee was more alert. The bad news: His recurring hernia had grown, and it was causing him significant pain. He also appeared to have an eye infection. While Becky and I were texting about these issues, she mentioned that Lee hadn't slept at all the night before. All of a sudden, a light bulb came on for me. Lee had been "time traveling" for a while now, believing it was decades earlier, thinking that he was on active military duty, asking about his mother, getting shocked at his older appearance when he looked in a mirror, and wanting to drink coffee all day long.

"Becky, Lee worked alternating shifts as a meteorologist during his twenties and thirties, often working the graveyard shift. Could the fact that he worked shifts back then and that he's been time traveling recently have some effect on his sleep patterns now?" I asked.

She immediately fired back, "Oh my gosh! I never consid-ered that he might have worked shifts as a weather forecaster! He definitely could be trying to return to his sleep patterns from decades ago!"

She explained that with terminal restlessness, it's not uncommon for people to revert to the sleep patterns of their younger years. This was bad news for the night caregivers and Lee. We might never get his days and nights straight.

By mid-October, Lee would have times when he'd become very disoriented, when his speech wasn't understandable at all. He would string together unrelated words that were un-intelligible. When that happened, I knew that he hadn't slept much the night before. Night-shift caregivers let me know that during some nights, he slept twenty minutes at a time, and those twenty minutes of sleep weren't very often.

NOVEMBER 2018

At the beginning of November, Taylor came up to me in the living room as I was walking through with Lee. I could tell by her body language that she was not happy. Taylor pulled no punches, getting right to the point, telling me, "Lee is insisting that Addie keep him company from the moment she gets into work for her shift at 4:00 a.m. He stands or sits at the kitchen counter for hours and insists that she talk with him and give him her full attention. The situation is stressing her out, and it's affecting the food service."

I didn't know what to say at first, but it made sense that if Lee was desperate to have someone with him during the early-morning hours, he'd turn to Addie when she arrived at 4:00 a.m. She had always chatted with Lee and Mich in the morn-ings before breakfast as she set the tables. She was friendly with everyone and obviously cared about Lee. He now refused to accept that she couldn't carry on a one-on-one conversation instead of working in the kitchen.

I had no solutions to offer. "I've known that Lee is not sleeping, hanging out in the living room at 3:00 or 4:00 a.m., but I had no idea that he is impacting Addie's or the other staff's ability to work. I'm so sorry."

Taylor explained, rapid-fire, that Lee was requiring much more time and care than any other resident. I could tell that she had reached her limit with the impact of his care. I felt my face flush in reaction to her tone, feeling as if I was being called on the carpet for Lee's actions even though I had no control over what he did. I did understand the dilemma Taylor faced. Lee was a beloved member of her McMillan "family," but his agitation, demands, and medical issues were sucking the life out of Taylor and the staff. Lee was already being charged the maximum rate possible, so she couldn't hire any more staff to deal with the workload issue.

Finally, Taylor gave me the bad news I'd been expecting for months: "You know that I care deeply about Lee and that we all love him here. But when his issues start affecting the care we give to other residents, I just can't ignore the situation."

That was it. Lee was going to be moved out of McMillan. My heart sank.

But then Taylor added, "So, I'm letting you know that the only way Lee can stay at McMillan is if you hire sitters twenty-four seven to keep him occupied."

I knew that chances were slim to none I could find sitters, but at least Taylor left the door open for Lee to stay at McMillan. I responded that I would get sitters right away.

The minute I arrived home, I called the caregiving agency that I had used before Lee moved into McMillan and learned that they didn't have enough available staff. I frantically called every agency in the valley and then called Jerri, fighting back tears about the situation. She knew everyone in the business.

Maybe she knew of an agency I hadn't tried? Jerri offered to see if she could drum up some help. A few hours later, she called back, letting me know that she'd found only one agency with a caregiver available every day, and only from 6:00 a.m. to 10:00 a.m. I called the agency supervisor and booked the time slot. Then I called Taylor to propose that I hire the agency's sitters for the 6:00 a.m. to 10:00 a.m. period and then take over myself, daily, from 10:00 a.m. until 9:00 p.m. I couldn't believe my ears when she agreed to this arrangement, even though Addie would have to make do from 4:00 a.m. until 6:00 a.m. and the night shift would be on their own. Taylor really did care about Lee; I knew the sacrifice she was making for him. The requirement for me to be at the facility wasn't too much of a change—I had been spending big chunks of my days there anyway, knowing that there wasn't much time left with Lee. I went to Addie and apologized for the situation and implored her to ignore Lee during the 4:00 a.m. to 6:00 a.m. hours, even if he got upset. I could tell from her eyes that it was going to be torture.

As the weeks of November passed, Lee's condition completely deteriorated. It was shocking to be able to sense his spirit slipping away. When I looked at his face and into his eyes, he didn't look back at me; his face and eyes were blank, as if the essence of my husband was missing.

Lee was completely disoriented now. For example, he performed nonsensical actions over and over. One day, he lifted his hand to his mouth like he was taking a sip from a cup of coffee, but there was no cup in his hand. I'd get him water with a straw and hold it for him, but he didn't want to actually suck on the straw or take a drink from a cup, only to act like he was. He became very confused, nonstop.

On November 23, Lee's swallowing difficulties got worse. He was starting to choke when he first tried to eat a few bites.

He was already on a smooth-foods diet, so there was nothing more that could be done.

On November 24, Lee began sleeping nearly all of the time and didn't want to eat more than a bite or two during each meal. Becky told me that these were the most common signs that the end was near and hugged me as we watched Lee resting.

On November 27, Lee was very weak and didn't talk much. He lay back in his recliner with his eyes closed, except when he needed to go to the bathroom three or four times that day. In order to get him there, I had to use a gait belt and hold it tightly to lift and guide him. By doing so, Lee could balance well enough to stand up and lean on the walker as he made his way. I remember being grateful that he could at least get himself to and from the restroom.

CHAPTER 11

The Last Days

NOVEMBER 29

When I entered McMillan first thing in the morning on November 29, I walked straight to Lee's room, as always. I found him still lying in bed, which was unusual. A couple of caregivers were standing next to the bed with concerned looks on their faces. These caregivers immediately told me that Lee could no longer stand and support his own weight. It was as if his lower body was out of his control. He was completely bedridden now.

The meaning of the words I'd just heard couldn't sink in at first. It was as if I couldn't understand English and struggled to make sense of what the caregivers had just said. Even though I should have expected this turn of events, my stomach pitched at the news. Once I grasped what I'd been told, I pulled up a chair next to the bed and took hold of Lee's hand.

Midmorning, Lee suddenly became extremely agitated and alert, demanding that he go to the bathroom and struggling to get out of bed. The caregivers and I tried to explain to him that he was too weak to get up. We implored him to go in his incontinence underwear and explained in every way possible that we would change the underwear immediately after he went. It seemed like Lee couldn't understand, or it just felt too foreign for him to lie there and go. Then he started loudly begging me to help him get to the bathroom. After about five minutes of his pleas, I couldn't stand it.

Moving the walker next to the bed, I pulled Lee to a sitting position and began to lift him up to the walker. Obviously, I wasn't thinking straight, not understanding that his legs couldn't support his weight or imagining that I could lift his dead weight myself. As I struggled, the three caregivers who were in the room at that time immediately jumped in to help. By the time we got him a couple of feet away from the bed, reality hit me. We were literally carrying Lee. After a considerable struggle moving across the room, we then couldn't get him seated on the toilet. It seemed as if his body below the waist was paralyzed. We had to manually bend his torso in order to get him seated. After finally arranging his body on the toilet, I realized he couldn't urinate on demand now. His lower body was completely out of his control.

The situation was dangerous for us all as we carried Lee back to bed. All I could do was apologize profusely and feel horrible for putting the caregivers through that. It was as if I had needed visual proof that Lee had reached the end. After we got him settled back in bed, we all broke down, group-hugging and crying. Lee never asked to go to the bathroom again.

My husband's Alzheimer's diagnosis had given me nine years' notice that this day would arrive, yet the situation still seemed surreal. Each and every time I left to get something from the kitchen or to go into the bathroom myself and then reentered the bedroom, I was shaken to see Lee lying helplessly in bed. That vision sent emotional shock waves throughout my body every time.

Lee was never fully conscious again, except for a handful of five-minute episodes when he opened his eyes and spoke. A few times, he just called my name, wanting to hold my hand. At one point, Lee was able to tell me that he needed me to be there with him, which cemented my resolve to stay by his side.

During one of these moments of unusual alertness, I knew that Lee sensed that he was gravely ill when he confided to me that he was afraid he wasn't good enough to go to heaven. I became solely focused on trying to help Lee find some peace and called our clergyman, who had visited him nearly every day over the last two weeks. I urgently asked for help finding Bible passages that would reassure Lee. Once I had a short list and hung up, I read the recommended passages slowly, out loud. Lee seemed more at ease and nodded with eyes closed when I asked if he believed that Jesus had died for his sins and that he would go to heaven. Then I played his favorite classical piano music at a very low volume. Eventually, I just sat quietly by Lee's side, holding his hand.

It was very hard for me to be away from Lee's room at all now. I worried that he'd look for me and not find me there. I went home as late at night as possible and wolfed down a bowl of oatmeal before I left the house as early as possible the next morning. I just sat next to the bed, holding Lee's hand and watching his face, from early morning until late at night, wanting to be sure he knew he wasn't alone. Two or three times, I left the room for a break, but I always felt drawn back to Lee's room within a couple of minutes. The hours blended into each other and seemed to pass quickly.

DECEMBER 1 AND 2

Lee woke up only three or four times during December 1 and 2. When he did, he squeezed my hand and asked if I was beside him. Shockingly, during two of those waking periods, he became unusually lucid. Lee talked so cogently, it was almost as if he weren't sick anymore, like the clock had been turned back ten years. Those two periods were eerie, as if I were witnessing a miracle.

During the first of the two awake periods, Lee talked about his life's regrets . . . that he hadn't felt comfortable spending money to travel as much as he now wished we had. It was a mistake, he said. And then Lee talked about his parenting hindsight, that he had been too strict with all of his children but most of all with his younger son. Lee said he was so grateful that, despite his parenting mistakes, this son had turned out to be a respectable, loving man. Lee also felt badly that he had lived out of the country for most of his adult life, so his parents rarely got to see him and their grandchildren. Once it seemed that Lee had run out of energy to say anything more, I reassured him that he was only human, that we all have our faults and all make mistakes, and that I was certain that he was dearly loved by all of his family and friends regardless. And God loved him, too, despite any sins he might have committed, I added. He smiled up at me and seemed to relax.

Hours later, during a second lucid period, I was given a most precious gift when Lee told me how much he loved me, in a way that took me back to our courtship. He seemed to speak straight from his heart.

At the end, he asked me, "If you had it to do all over again, would you marry me?"

I was shocked by the question, then realized that he needed to know that he was a good husband. Answering without any hesitation, hoping he could sense my authenticity, I said, "Yes,

yes, yes, Lee. I would marry you again in a heartbeat. You have been the husband I always wanted and needed, because you've always made sure that I know deep down to my core that you love me, and no one else has ever done that. Yes, Lee, I would marry you again. I love you even more today than I did the day I married you."

The whole time I spoke, he smiled up at me with those blue eyes. It was almost as if the Alzheimer's had disappeared for just a few minutes. Before he closed his eyes again, Lee told me that he didn't know what he would have done without me; he thanked me for always being by his side and for caring for him in the way I had. I knew that these words would carry me for the rest of my life and worked hard to hang on to them, to never forget them.

Lee seemed visibly relaxed after he closed his eyes this time. The fact that he was able to communicate so eloquently on his deathbed reinforced my belief that God does exist. It didn't make sense to me that he was so weak that he had barely been able to form words earlier and yet he now had initiated this thoughtful conversation with me. As I sat by his bed, holding his hand, I reflected on the character and strength of the man I'd fallen in love with and the miracle of meeting him completely by chance.

Lee appeared to be sleeping deeply now and didn't wake up when someone spoke in the room or even when his underwear was changed.

On the afternoon of December 2, I saw a new, weird sore on Lee's back when I helped a caregiver change him. It was bright red, near his tailbone. When I showed this sore to Becky, she was silent for a few minutes. Then she took me into the hallway and explained that it was a Kennedy ulcer, which required special care. Caring for the ulcer would require sterile gloves and bandages for cleansing, a special medicated cream, and frequent checks. If not treated properly, it could be extremely painful.

"Patients develop a Kennedy ulcer when their circulatory system can no longer provide sufficient oxygen and nutrients for the body's skin needs," she explained. "The skin is our largest organ and the first to let us know when the body can no longer sustain itself, kind of like the canary in a coal mine. In the vast majority of my cases, patients haven't lived for more than three days after a Kennedy ulcer first appeared."

I knew that Lee was near the end, but seeing concrete proof of that was still a shock . . . every single time.

Hospice nurse Amy placed Lee on a set schedule of morphine drops to combat the pain of the Kennedy ulcer. If Lee became agitated or grimaced or fidgeted in bed, the med tech had a set order that allowed her to administer drops without any other authorization, up to a pre-set maximum. They tried to keep the dosage as low as possible so that he could communicate, if able.

During the prior week, I had tried to feed Lee anything I could think of that he might be able to swallow and digest—scrambled eggs, yogurt, cream of wheat, soup. Addie and Becky tried, too. The cooks gave me free rein in the kitchen and pantry to make whatever I thought he needed late at night. Lee would only eat one or two bites of scrambled eggs and nothing else I offered. Then, on December 2, Lee completely stopped eating everything. When I tried giving him Ensure, he refused that, too. Becky explained to me that his entire system was shutting down and that at this point, he wouldn't be able to digest anything. If I were able to somehow get him to eat a few bites, he would just vomit it back up because his stomach and bowels were no longer functioning. I stopped trying to coax him into eating.

Soon after, I realized that Lee couldn't swallow drinks either. So, Becky gave me a special aid for this situation, a Popsicle-looking stick that had a small square sponge attached to the end. She had me soak the sponge in a glass of clean water.

When I laid the sponge end on his tongue and pressed a little, he swallowed the drips of water that dribbled into his mouth and would even occasionally suck water out of the sponge, all while he looked asleep.

I stayed by Lee's side as much as possible now, only going home for a short nap and shower. I absolutely did not want my husband dying alone.

DECEMBER 3

On December 3, Lee could no longer swallow at all. When I put the sponge swab on his tongue, he choked if any water dribbled down his throat. Becky and Logan tried, too, and he choked for them as well. His body had shut down completely. I knew that he couldn't live for long without water. Lee slept peacefully. I sat next to the bed and held his hand. The hours passed in a fog.

DECEMBER 4

On December 4, I left for home at around 6:30 p.m. to grab a bite to eat and a nap. Right after I walked in the door at home, an inescapable feeling deep in my gut hit me like a huge wave. I had this urgent feeling that I needed to get back to Lee. Not more than ten minutes later, I walked back into his room to find that the situation had completely changed. Lee had been peacefully sleeping just twenty minutes earlier but now was distraught, stretching his arms up from his prone body as far as they could reach, almost raising his head up off the bed, as he tried to touch the corner of the ceiling opposite the head of the bed. He was talking to his late mother when his eyes popped open as he blankly searched the ceiling.

This scene was frightening to me. But soon after I sat down, my panic faded as I remembered reading that reaching for the ceiling and talking to deceased family members was a common occurrence just before death. And then I remembered the time when a resident's door across the hall from Lee's room was quickly opened as I happened to walk by, and as I glanced in that direction, I had seen a lady doing the same thing, on the day before she died.

Lee looked distraught as he strained to reach for the sky. I had never heard or read about the best actions to take when this happened or even what to do in general when someone was in the process of dying. I had no idea what would be best for Lee's sake at this point and felt I was winging it. After praying on what to do, I felt I needed to take guidance from Lee, when he had asked me to sit by him and hold his hand. I reached under the covers and gently grasped one of his hands to see what would happen. I figured he could always let go of my hand if this wasn't the right thing to do. Lee squeezed my hand, tightly, and never let go. Holding hands seemed to calm him some, although he was still stretching toward the ceiling with his other hand.

Becky came into the room to check on Lee, and when she saw him reaching up toward the ceiling with his right arm, she told me that it wouldn't be long now. After three or so hours, Lee dropped his arm and got very still. He didn't open his eyes or move around ever again but did continue to squeeze my hand. It was as if my entire being was focused on our clasped hands now, on the fact that his hand was the only connection I had to Lee and my hand was the only connection he had to this world. It struck me that everything in his body was shutting down except for this one hand that gripped mine. I just couldn't let go. At around 3:00 a.m., too exhausted to sit up any longer, I pushed Lee's recliner up against his bed, lay back in it, then took hold of Lee's hand again. He tightly gripped mine right back. We held hands, lying parallel and with our upper arms pressed against each other, and slept. When I woke up three hours later, we were still holding hands.

DECEMBER 5

I sat up in the recliner at around 6:30 a.m. When I did, Lee's grip relaxed and no longer held my hand. I moved the chair away from the bed, and Becky checked his vitals.

She warned, "His breathing will become shallow, and possibly irregular, and may even stop every now and then. This is the end. I'm so sorry."

She checked his fingers and feet to see if they had turned dark blue or purple, a sign that death was imminent. They hadn't. Becky gave me a hug as she left the room. I pulled out a little pocket Bible to read some Psalms but couldn't concentrate.

By that afternoon, I couldn't stop myself from staring at Lee's breathing as it became more shallow and less regular. He would stop breathing for what seemed like minutes and then breathe more regularly again for a little while. Finally, at 9:00 p.m., Lee drew a shallow breath for the last time.

The lead night-shift caregiver informed Amy. Once she came and pronounced Lee's death, she called the funeral home I had chosen so they could retrieve Lee's body before the other residents woke up in the morning. I wanted badly to be with Lee as he was carried out, but I just couldn't make it past midnight and left before the funeral-home staff arrived. My body gave in to the numbing fatigue that washed over me.

DECEMBER 6

Trembling in the cold, while trying to see through the scraped portions of my windshield that revealed a striped view of the road between streaks of ice, I steered my car through the pitch-black first hour of the day. Mine was the only car on the road to home. It felt as if I truly were the only person on earth. With no people on the sidewalks, no cars on the street, and now without Lee in my world, I was as alone as one could be. That realization was terrifying, and tears began streaming down my face.

Yet at the same time, I had an overwhelming urge to lift up prayers of thanksgiving. I felt compelled to thank God out loud, because Lee's passing was not painful. During his last days, the staff had made it their mission to be sure this was true. While driving home, I tried to think of a way I could repay Becky, Taylor, and all of the staff at McMillan for the way they had lovingly cared for Lee (and me) throughout the last two and a half years. Lee and I couldn't have survived without them. I also felt compelled to praise God for guiding me through so many challenges over all of the years of Lee's illness. And, finally, recalling Lee's last words to me, I thanked God and my dear husband out loud for that last gift he had given to me: peace.

EPILOGUE

It's been over four years, and my brain fog and forgetfulness, which seemed permanent during Lee's last months and after his death, have cleared up. The constant pit in my stomach is gone, too. Yet it still occasionally feels odd that all of my time is my own. I will never stop missing the sound of Lee's voice or the sparkle of his blue eyes.

I have to admit now that while decision-making as a caregiver felt pretty straightforward when I cared for Lee at home, decisions were much more difficult once he moved into the memory-care facility. I felt drawn to visit every day so he wouldn't feel abandoned. I also felt compelled more and more as time passed to try and distract Lee, to keep the agitation at bay. Yet at times, my presence frustrated him because I refused to take him home. The lack of a clear answer on the best approach created a real quandary. In the end, Lee let me know on his deathbed what had been most important to him: that I had been there at his side.

I wish that Lee's last years had been easier on him emotionally and physically, but I have to be grateful that he was never in real pain, thanks to excellent medical care. And, although dementia definitely affected his quality of life, it didn't affect the basic essence of who Lee was. My husband still found joy in car rides out in the country, in spending time with friends and family, in travel, in supporting his Boise State Broncos football team, in savoring his much-loved frozen yogurt . . .

and in the simple joy of watching cloud formations in the sky. The Alzheimer's also didn't prevent Lee from showing me in many small ways that he still loved me. I will always be grateful for the years we had together after his diagnosis.

If you are actively caregiving, please remind yourself daily to trust in your intrinsic knowledge and skills, to believe in your gut instincts, to recognize and accept when other people have the desire and ability to help you, and to ignore the unavoidable, incurable critics. I sincerely hope that you will sense, as I did, that God is always by your side.

Do not be anxious about anything, but in every situation, by prayer and petition, with thanksgiving, present your requests to God. And the peace of God, which transcends all understanding, will guard your hearts and your minds in Christ Jesus. Philippians 4:6–7

ADL Assessment

Choose the number of the description that is closest to how well your loved one manages his or her own activities. Write that score on the blank at left. Add the scores.

Your loved one:

_____ **Meals**

3 can prepare his or her own nutritious meals if needed
2 can prepare simple meals, like a sandwich or cereal, but not cook a full meal
2 makes occasional poor meal choices at times
1 is unable to prepare any nutritious meals, needs someone to serve meals to him/her

_____ **Eating**

3 feeds self, cuts meat, chews and swallows without trouble
2 needs help to cut up food or needs help feeding
1 is at significant risk of choking, either with solids or liquids, or eats much less than before and is losing weight

_____ **Toilet**

3 needs no help or is able to independently toilet with the
   help of grab bars
2 needs assistance with pulling up or down clothing or with
   wiping, or has occasional accidents
1 is incontinent, needs to wear adult incontinence underwear, or needs help with all toileting tasks

_____ **Mobility**

3 has not fallen in the past six months, does not need assistance walking outside or inside
2 has an occasional fall, needs help outside, or needs the help
   of a walker
1 is not able to support weight on legs or not able to walk,
   needs a wheelchair to get around

_____ **Transfer**

3 independently moves from sitting or lying to standing (or
   needs rare assistance)
2 always needs one person's assistance moving from sitting
   or lying to standing
1 can't stand or support his or her own body weight or needs
   two-person assistance to get out of a bed or chair

_____ **Hygiene**

3   independently shaves, combs hair, and brushes teeth without reminders
2   needs some reminders or assistance almost daily with hair, shaving, or toothbrushing
1   is dependent on others for toothbrushing, hair combing, shaving, etc.

_____ **Bathing**

3   can bathe on his or her own at least two times a week without reminders, assistance, or supervision
2   needs assistance, cueing, reminders, or occasional help with bathing or shampooing
1   doesn't know how to bathe and shampoo, even after receiving help to a shower chair

_____ **Transportation**

3   can drive or use public transportation on his or her own without issues
2   is starting to have problems with their driving skills or using public transit or Uber or Lyft, or is getting lost
1   is dependent on others to drive or needs ambulance for transportation

_____ **Dressing**

3 selects clothing (even if mismatched) and independently dresses or undresses
2 needs reminders, info about weather-appropriate clothing, or occasional help dressing or undressing
1 is completely dependent on others for getting dressed or undressed

_____ **Finances**

3 independently manages finances, pays own bills, or needs only occasional assistance
2 makes occasional errors with financial transactions or tracking finances or has lost card once
1 is unable to manage finances or pay bills; or has had a check returned or a debit or credit card transaction denied; or has lost credit cards often

_____ **Shopping**

3 can effectively create a shopping list, find needed items, and shop without assistance
2 needs reminders, supervision, or assistance with list-making or shopping
1 is totally dependent upon others for shopping

_____ **Laundry**

3 maintains a supply of clean clothes in passable condition
2 needs reminders, help, or supervision washing, drying, and folding laundry
1 is dependent on others for laundry services

_____ **Nighttime**

3 needs no help during the night
2 needs help during the night on average up to once a week
1 needs someone available multiple times a week or more

_____ **Emergencies**

3 would recognize and evacuate or call 911 if any emergency
   arose
2 would need help recognizing an emergency, but could
   assist in getting help
1 requires someone to recognize an emergency, call for help,
   and help evacuate if necessary

_____ **Medications**

3 can manage ordering supply of medications, tracking dosages, and self-administering on time
2 needs cueing or help managing and ordering refills or
   needs other supervision
1 is totally dependent upon others for medication purchasing, tracking, and administration

_____ **Activities**

3 is able to independently manage social activities, hobbies,
   or other enjoyed activities
2 needs some help to arrange or supervise activities, or fre-
   quently says he/she is bored
1 requires daily oversight, planned activities, or diversions,
   or is depressed or has outbursts

_____ **Equipment**

3 uses only dentures, glasses, CPAP, contacts, or hearing-aid equipment
2 needs a cane or walker to get around
1 requires a wheelchair to get around or requires oxygen supply

_____ **Support**

3 has family member, friend, church member, or social worker help dependably at least three times a week
2 has family member, friend, church member, or social worker help occasionally
1 has no help

_____ **Housework**

3 is able to vacuum/sweep, clean bathrooms, dust, and change sheets at least twice a month (plus #2)
2 can keep kitchen counters and tables clean, change out toilet-paper rolls, take out trash
1 is unable to do any housekeeping on his or her own

_____ **TOTAL**

SCORING (The lowest score is 19—someone needing the most help; the highest score is 57—an independent person)

50–57: A person who is completely independent
40–49: A person who needs some help
30–39: A person who needs significant help
19–29: A person who is completely dependent on others

ABOUT THE AUTHOR

Donna Larkin is a former public affairs writer who earned a master's degree in education and distance learning. This educational background instilled in her a problem-solving approach to every challenge she has taken on, including caregiving. She grew up in a suburb of New York City and lived in San Francisco and Los Angeles for eight years before establishing a home in Idaho to raise her family. Donna and her husband, Lee, had nearly twenty-five blessed years together before he passed away of Alzheimer's disease in 2018.